e

e

The Work of the Parish Church Nurse

Julia Quiring-Emblen

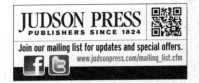

The Work of the Parish Church Nurse

© 2014 by Judson Press, Valley Forge, PA 19482-0851

All rights reserved.

Judson Press has made every effort to trace the ownership of all quotes. In the event of a question arising from the use of a quote, we regret any error made and will be pleased to make the necessary correction in future printings and editions of this book.

Interior design by Wendy Ronga, Hampton Design Group.

Cover design by Danny Ellison.

Library of Congress Cataloging-in-Publication data

Quiring-Emblen, Julia. The work of the parish church nurse/Julia Quiring-Emblen.—First edition. pages cm

ISBN 978-0-8170-1740-8 (pbk.: alk. paper) 1. Parish nursing. 2. Pastoral medicine. I. Title. RT120.P37E43 2014 610.73—dc23

2013026097

Printed in the U.S.A.

First Edition, 2014.

CONTENTS

PREFACE

Theologian Martin Marty once asked a church leader for advice concerning a person who had just received bad medical news. The church leader responded: "My advice is that the person should have been an active member of a vital congregation for quite a few years." Marty explained that such a congregation would enfold the person in intercessory prayer and provide cards, casseroles, and visits.[1] This has been the church's traditional response to the illness of members as the institutional church has established itself all over the U.S.

Since Jesus healed people during his earthly ministry, his disciples continued to provide care for the sick to promote healing when possible. Returning to a strong church focus on a healing ministry is not only following Christ's model, but it is also needful because of the current economics of healthcare and limited availability of medical personnel. The work of the parish nurse in the church provides concern for the sick and promotion of health for the members of the congregation and the surrounding community.

What is a parish nurse? A parish nurse is a licensed nurse, typically with church office space in which to work and to talk with members of the congregation, who focuses on the integration of the church beliefs regarding faith and healing with the medical science of treating illness and promoting health. This book is designed to illustrate how Christ's healing work can be extended by the work of the parish nurse.

You may have some of the following questions:

- We have a congregation, not a parish! What is a parish nurse?
- How might a nurse start working at church?
- Why might a nurse be needed to work at a church?
- If two individuals are both church members and registered nurses, how does the work of the parish nurse differ from another's nursing work (e.g., in a doctor's office, hospital, or assisted living center)?

The succeeding chapters answer these and other questions about the religious background of the church in healthcare, specific preparation for parish nurses, organization and accountability in the parish nurse ministry, and specific ministry tasks undertaken by the parish nurse on Sunday and throughout the week. One chapter also addresses the role of the parish nurse in Christian outreach.

Throughout this volume, we will consider the ministries of four fictional parish nurses: Mary, Nina, Dolores, and Jake. Their ministries are based in part on the author's own experiences and on anecdotal comments shared by other parish nurses. Their stories are designed to illustrate to members of a congregation what a parish nurse at work in a local church might accomplish. Examples of materials are developed in the chapters and others are presented as appendices at the back of the book and materials available online so that nurses in a congregation might adapt and use them if or when they move into a parish nurse role.

Notes

1. Martin E. Marty, "Introduction" in *Parish Nursing*, ed. Phyllis Ann Solari-Twadell and Mary Ann McDermott (Thousand Oaks, CA: Sage Publications, 1999), xx.

ACKNOWLEDGMENTS

I would like to thank Glenna Stewart, a nurse friend, for reading an early draft and offering very helpful suggestions. Claudia Bagley has provided me with computer assistance—helping me organize materials and managing chapter details.

I would especially like to thank my mother, Marianna Quiring, for helping me arrange time to write, answering the phone, and encouraging me to write so points and examples are clear to the readers.

The Judson Press editorial staff has been most helpful in clarifying points and ideas that made the process of writing and revising proceed smoothly.

CHAPTER 1

Historical Perspective

The role that religion and the church have played in providing care comes from a long historical tradition. As far back as 400 and 300 BC, Greek and Roman temples were involved in health and were known as places of healing. The old Greek Hippocratic Oath reflects care for the sick. Hippocrates and other physicians during this period divided the body into parts such as circulatory, pulmonary, and gastrointestinal systems. This made it simpler to study and care for specific systems or areas of the body, rather than focusing on the needs of the whole person.

The Old Testament laws include concern for health needs, such as prohibitions against eating certain animals because they were "unclean." The washing and cleansing rituals may now be understood to foreshadow Christ's cleansing us from sin, but they also reflect concern for health issues. Consider that hand-washing may have been even more important to health in ancient times compared to the present day, when water, sinks, and good soaps are so readily available in many countries.

Jesus initiated healing as a way to demonstrate his power. He miraculously healed physical problems, such as paralysis and disease, and performed mental and emotional healing by casting out evil spirits and forgiving sins. Through the centuries his apostles and followers have continued to assist in healing work using physical touch by laying on hands and praying. The early church congregations sent deacons (male and female) into homes to bathe and feed the ill and dying, applying whatever treatments were available at the time.

Phoebe, a female deacon identified in Romans 16:1-2, provides a model for working with the poor and the needy. As the church grew during this time, some of the widows and matrons established places of comfort for the ill. Deacon Fabiola sold her possessions and used her own funds to care for the sick and the poor. Because of this work she is credited in history for establishing the first Roman hospital for the poor in AD 300.[1]

At that time hospitals were primarily places where people were brought to die. Without the availability and use of many disinfectants and antibiotics, those who were already ill often contracted an infectious disease from another patient and that new infection caused their death. Knowing that hospitals were hothouses of incubation for infectious diseases, people with funds cared for ill family members at home by hiring persons to come into their homes to provide basic care—feeding, bathing, and washing wounds.

In the Middle Ages the Christian church and selected people associated with it provided care for the sick. Typically monks and nuns were involved in a healing ministry, often staffing places of care for the ill. The long and bloody Crusades required more development of care for those injured in battle. Some monks and nuns traveled with the military groups while others set up places to care for the injured. Gradually members of monasteries and convents established hospitals, and a healing ministry with hospitals became part of their building complex. Some of the hospitals were called "lazarettos" after Lazarus, the brother of Mary and Martha, whom Jesus brought back to life (John 11:43-44).[2]

In the 1600s Descartes philosophized about the dualism of body and spirit, and for a time this view deterred the church from focusing on physical healing. Medicine focused on care for the physical body, while care for the broken spirit was left for the clergy.[3]

During the 1700s and 1800s, with civilization moving west in the New World, churches were also established and women's groups in these churches began to provide for the needs of the sick and poor by setting up clinics and then hospitals. Many hospitals (such as Lutheran General Hospital in Park Ridge, Illinois) and medical centers (such as Emanuel Medical Center (Lutheran) and Adventist Medical Center, both in Portland, Oregon) still reflect some of the church influence in their names. The deaconess movement became a strong influence in establishing Protestant hospitals while Catholic sisters established hospitals with names like "Providence" and "Sacred Heart."

While working as a hospital chaplain at what is now the University of Chicago Medical Center, clergyman Granger Westberg began to realize that many illnesses had a spiritual origin and found that patients did not respond well when treatment was only physical. In 1976 he began working with others to establish health centers for the "whole" person, which were family doctors' offices located in churches.

Granger Westberg deliberately chose the term *wholistic* to distinguish these health centers from standard medical care. At the inaugural Westberg Institute in 1982, Westberg explained why he chose the term *wholistic*: to represent "wholeness" of body, mind, and spirit provided in a faith community. He sensed that what is termed *holistic* medicine went beyond traditional American medicine because it included alternative therapies. He kept in close contact with the American Medical Association, the Association of American Medical Colleges, and bishops and officers of mainline churches, all of which encouraged innovation as long as it was within reasonable limits.[4]

Some of these Wholistic Health Centers were sponsored by the W. K. Kellogg Foundation and the Department of Preventive Medicine and Community Health at the University of Illinois College of Medicine. With the financial backing of these groups, Westberg and others helped set up more than a dozen medical clinics located in churches of different socioeconomic levels throughout the country. Such clinics included physicians, nurses, laboratory personnel, social workers, and other healthcare personnel.[5]

Maintaining these clinics became costly and difficult when grant funds ran out. After careful evaluation of clinic activities, one finding stood out: The nurse was the glue that bound the physician and the clergy together. Because the nurses spoke both the scientific and religious languages, they served as effective translators clarifying information between clergy and patients, physicians and patients, and clergy and physicians.[6]

In 1985 Westberg and his supporting committee sponsored a group of six nurses who worked in different churches and came together at Lutheran General Hospital in Park Ridge, Illinois, one morning a week to talk about their nursing experiences. Through these discussions it became apparent that nurses were in the best position to encourage preventive medicine. People talked to the nurse about their concerns prior to going to the doctor. If the nurse could help to identify potential problems early, steps could be put in place to effectively prevent illness or disease.[7]

As the preventive aspect expanded, sick care gradually changed to the promotion of wellness activities that offset illness. As the nurses worked in the church context, they also included spiritual care, building bridges between the medical and church communities by facilitating care focused on the needs of the whole person.

Westberg and his supporters recognized that persons coming to church to worship are whole people, not only spirits and not only bodies. Persons entering the church doors bring their broken legs, ulcers, or other illnesses along with them to the worship service. The needs of the whole person must be considered in spiritual and physical healing.

Because of Westberg's work, the National Parish Nurse Resource Center (NPNRC) was established in 1986. The first annual Westberg Symposium was held in 1987 to bring nurses together to discuss topics related to Parish Nursing. The NPNRC became the International Parish Nurse Resource Center (IPNRC) and moved from Park Ridge,

Illinois, to St. Louis, Missouri, in 2002. In 2011 headquarters for the IPNRC moved to Memphis, Tennessee, where it now functions as part of the Church Health Center (www.parishnurses.org).[8]

According to the the International Parish Nurse Resource Center, the mission of parish nursing is stated as

> ...the intentional integration of the practices of faith and nursing so that people can achieve wholeness in, with, and through the community of faith in which serve.[9]

Questions

1. How do members of your congregation view health?
2. To whom do they turn when illness symptoms surface?
3. How is the traditional healing ministry of the church carried out in your church?
4. How might the traditional healing ministry be enhanced in your congregation?
5. In your church, what do you think would be the most important steps to take in order to prevent disease and promote health for the whole person?

Notes

1. L. James Wylie and Phyllis Ann Solari-Twadell, "Health and the Congregation," in *Parish Nursing*, ed. Phyllis Ann Solari-Twadell and Mary Ann McDermott (Thousand Oaks, CA: Sage Publications, 1999), 26.

2. C. Scherzer, "The Church and Healing" (unpublished manuscript, 1984), Deaconess Hospital, Evansville, IN.

3. L. James Wylie and Phyllis Ann Solari-Twadell.

4. William M. Peterson, "Granger Westberg Verbatim: A Vision for Faith and Health," published for the inaugural of the Westberg Institute in 1982 and reprinted by the IPNRC: St Louis, 2002, under the title "Wholistic and Holistic," 43.

5. D. Tubesing, "An Idea in Evolution," in *History of the Wholistic Health Centers Project* (Hinsdale, IL: Society for Wholistic Medicine, 1977).

6. Granger Westberg, "A Personal Historical Perspective of Whole Person Health and the Congregation," in *Parish Nursing*, ed. Phyllis Ann Solari-Twadell and Mary Ann McDermott (Thousand Oaks, CA: Sage Publications, 1999), 35.

7. Ibid., 37–38.

8. IPNRC address: 1210 Peabody Ave., Memphis, TN 38104; IPNRC website: https://www.facebook.com/pages/International-Parish-Nurse-Resource-Center-IPNRC/193648440675125.

9. See "About: Mission" at www.parishnurses.org.

CHAPTER 2

Official Structure of Parish Nursing

This chapter explains the various names that may be used to refer to what is presented here as the parish nurse (PN). It designates key qualifications and the educational background of the PN. Some points pertaining to a job description are presented, along with five general roles and examples of each that indicate the kinds of activities most PNs engage in as they practice.

Alternative Names

Since a parish nurse role typically includes spiritual or religious dimensions, the title of a person selected to work with different religious denominations and groups becomes an important issue for each of the religious groups. According to Merriam-Webster's dictionary, the *parish* is the ecclesiastical unit of area committed to one pastor, with the residents of such an area, or the members of one church, also termed the *parish*. For example, in some Protestant groups the area surrounding the structure for worship is called the parish and the persons in the group are the parishioners. Roman Catholic institutions frequently refer to the area around their place of worship as their parish. For those who coined the phrase "parish nursing," the term *parish* was quite explicit. Adding the word *nurse* clarified the type of work that the person in the role was to do.

The name becomes less clear in Judaism because the person works in a local Hebrew synagogue rather than in a parish. So with some groups the term *faith community nurse* has been used to replace the *parish nurse* designation. In Islam, Hinduism, Buddhism, and in countries with other faith traditions, the *faith community* designation may also be more useful.

With the formation of the Health Ministries Association as a multidisciplinary, interfaith organization in 1989, another title, *health ministry nurse*, was designated. When groups differ in organization and focus, it often follows that the terms used to designate people change. The American Nurses Association (ANA), the accrediting group for professional nurses, tries to be sensitive and accommodate the needs of all working in the nursing field. *Faith community nursing* has become the designation used by the ANA for nurses working to integrate a health and wellness approach to the needs of persons.

For many, the original term *parish nurse* remains the clearest designation of the role, and so it continues as the name of choice for most in Protestant and Catholic church groups. The professional literature refers to Parish Nurse/Faith Community Nurse to illustrate that both of the terms are acceptable.[1]

Qualifications

As with every profession, parish nursing has requirements for standardized educational preparation, licensure, and practice activities. When Mountain View Church (name changed to maintain confidentiality) decided to hire a parish nurse for their congregation, a committee developed a list of the qualifications that were needed. The church's goal was to find someone in their congregation to become their nurse, if at all possible. The church board even said it would underwrite the cost of some specific training if a person was found without the parish nurse credentials.

The three qualifications in bold typeface in the following sample list of desired credentials *must* be in place before a person begins any work position designated as parish nurse.

- **Current nursing license in the state of practice**
- Baccalaureate nursing degree with three or more years of practice
- **Completion of basic standardized core curriculum endorsed by the International Parish Nurse Resource Center** (see "Curriculum" below)
- **Specialized knowledge of the religious beliefs and practices of the church denomination**
- Background in clinical pastoral education

Work experience or training related to interpersonal relationships and communication skills is recommended as well. Some experience working in community health as it relates to assessment of needs and specialized health and wellness programs is highly desirable. Continuing nursing education programs in clinical areas are also useful to maintain current clinical knowledge.

Curriculum for Parish Nurse Education

The foundational course designed by the International Parish Nurse Resource Center (IPNRC) prepares registered nurses for this specialty practice. The course consists of modules that are divided into the following units:

- Spirituality
- Professionalism
- Wholistic health
- Community

Topics include prayer, self-care, ethical issues, documentation, health promotion, life issues of violence, suffering and grief, assessment, and care coordination.

Current course information can be obtained from the IPNRC website.[2] In some areas there are geographical groups that can be contacted for information regarding local program offerings (such as Northwest Parish Nurse Ministries at www.npnm.org).

Each unit varies in length from two to four hours, for a composite total of thirty-one to thirty-six contact hours.

Job Description

In preparing to interview candidates, the Mountain View Church committee searched for a job description. They came to understand that though some resources identified what the parish nurse did in one church, the activities might be different in another.

L. J. Mayhugh and K. H. Martens reported on a study they conducted that asked the congregation what parish nurse services they preferred in their congregation.[3] In their survey they found that the highest ranked services were educational services pertaining to health screening, staying well, and emotional health. Nurse consultation about physical problems was another high preference. This congregational group also wanted the nurse to visit people after hospitalization and to visit the terminally ill.

An article by Rita P. Wilson indicated that parish nurses may support physical health and wellness by using health promotion and prevention activities.[4] She noted classes on wellness and exercise as examples. For the mind she suggested social support for the elderly dealing with loss and classes on stress as two key examples. Wilson indicated that the spiritual aspect should be interwoven along with physical and emotional aspects. Examples she cited include spiritual assessment, prayer, scripture reading, and discussion of religious issues relevant to care.

The Mountain View search committee members decided that their checklist of activities might include things the parish nurse does and does not do:

The Parish Nurse Does

Educate:

1. Conduct health screenings
2. Promote wellness
3. Assist with emotional health
4. Consult about physical problems
5. Visit people soon after hospitalization
6. Visit the terminally ill

Provide spiritual care:

7. Pray with people
8. Show compassion and caring
9. Discuss spiritual concerns during illness
10. Take Communion to the homebound (if accepted in church activities for non-deacons)

The Parish Nurse Does Not

1. Reject conventional medical and nursing science
2. Provide hands-on care
3. Share confidential health information
4. Become a substitute for healthcare

Additional Skills Useful in Parish Nursing:

1. Practice good organizational skills
2. Communicate effectively by demonstrating good interpersonal skills
3. Demonstrate good understanding of spiritual practice and religious knowledge and traditions of denomination and particular congregation
4. Work well independently and as a team member

General Parish Nurse Roles

Granger Westberg identified key areas of ministry for the parish nursing project.[5] These areas are reduced to five activities considered integral to the work of the active PN. Each is defined and then illustrated in the following anecdotes featuring four parish nurse models, Mary, Dolores, Nina, and Jake.

Health Educator. Upon assessing the needs of individuals and groups in the church community, the parish nurse decides on topics that may require individual teaching, become workshops, or be presented as group discussions. The parish nurse may teach Sunday school classes, present workshops, and design exercise classes. Experts may be called in to present special topics and for other assistance. The following illustration depicts this role.

After being employed for four months as a parish nurse at Mountain View (membership of 400), Mary decided to review her records. She found that she had talked with fifteen people regarding their questions about some aspect of dietary management related to illness. Several people came regarding their type 2 diabetes. Two men came because they were dealing with hypertension issues that were dietary-related. So she decided to offer a workshop focusing on key details of two common dietary concerns: sugar and salt. Inspired by an article titled "Shake Off the Salt," she decided to call the workshop "Cut the Sugar; Shake Off the Salt." (The workshop can be found at http://www.judsonpress.com/free_download_book_excerpts.cfm.)

Health Counselor. Persons make individual appointments to discuss a variety of needs, including personal and family issues with children. Often people come with issues related to surgical or medical treatments. The problems people want to discuss with the nurse in a calm, safe environment are often related to management of chronic disease.

Sometimes early intervention can prevent major health problems. An example of counseling regarding health follows.

In her tiny office at Mt. Zion African Methodist Episcopal (AME) Church, Dolores's next appointment was with a church member who had called to ask about how many pounds she could safely lose each week.

Evelyn arrived on time and was eager to talk. "My doctor told me to lose thirty pounds so my blood pressure might come down. I've been trying, but it is so hard. The children and my husband laugh at me when they have a regular meat-and-potatoes meal, and all I have to eat is some lettuce, cottage cheese, and a fruit plate."

"That is hard. Are you following a specific diet?" Dolores asked.

"No, the doctor told me all diets are about the same. She made some recommendations but said it didn't matter what I ate—except that I needed to eat less and lose weight," Evelyn explained.

Dolores knew the first step was for Evelyn's family to support her efforts. "Have you told your family about the doctor's recommendations?"

"Not exactly—I just said that I had to lose weight," Evelyn replied.

Dolores urged Evelyn to talk with her family more candidly. "They need to know about your blood pressure and how it is connected to your weight. Start with your husband; if your children see him being supportive, they will probably follow his example."

Dolores paused to pray with Evelyn that God would give her words to speak and prepare her husband and children to receive the news with compassion and eagerness to help. Then she and Evelyn consulted some resources to come up with a reasonable menu and a safe, conservative weight loss plan.

Not far away at Primera Iglesia Bautista Hispana, Nina met with Tomas to discuss getting additional help in caring for his wife, Carmen, at home. Carmen had only partial mobility following a stroke, and Tomas told Nina that he was at his wit's end.

"I know some people who care for their spouse for years and seem to enjoy it, but I guess I am not a very good husband. I can't get all the housework done and help Carmen in and out of bed and to the bathroom three to four times a day. Our teenaged granddaughter comes once a week and stays with her *abuela* while I get groceries. She tries to help with laundry or some cleaning while she's there." Tomas paused a moment to shake his head. "My work in the hardware store didn't prepare me for what I need to do now. I'm just so exhausted by it all."

"You are into very different kind of work now," Nina noted. "Do you use a lift or can Carmen help in transferring herself from bed to a chair?"

"We use a lift. A therapist comes three days a week to help her exercise," Tomas explained. "I help her do her exercises on the days the therapist doesn't come."

When she had a picture of what their day was like, Nina counseled Tomas about different types of assistance he might want to consider. Tomas decided that he really wanted someone to come three days a week to clean and cook some meals. He liked to do some of the cooking, but he just wanted a break.

Nina also recommended that Tomas look into a respite program for caregivers. "Caregivers need to have breaks to reenergize," Nina explained. "They offer some fun activities and small group sessions to share joys and struggles—and they serve good food! And it is free. I could arrange to get someone to take care of Carmen if you'd like to go."

"Sign me up, and also would you help me find someone to help with cooking and cleaning?" Tomas already sounded more energized at the prospect of more help.

Integrator of Faith and Health. The role of integrator of faith and health is essential for every PN. Such integration may take the form of praying with someone about a health concern, as Dolores did with Evelyn in the example above. It may involve offering biblical wisdom about issues of healthy lifestyles, be it in the form of physical health or mental and emotional well-being (see Jake's example below). It may also involve the even more challenging task of helping people think and pray through difficult health decisions that involve moral and ethical controversies.

Healthcare has become so secularized that people simply accept some of the directives from healthcare providers without considering faith issues. Some people put such great trust in suggested treatments that they blindly follow care directives until they are confronted with some threat to their well-being. Only when surgery is scheduled do they call the pastor to ask for prayer. In a sense, this is the Band-Aid approach.

Rather than struggle along with painful treatments and fear of the unknown, they could learn to integrate their faith on a daily basis as they personally turn to God for help. It may help people to receive some scriptural promises for peace as they learn to focus on God (Isaiah 26:3) rather than their fear. A verse such as Isaiah 30:15 tells us that we gain strength as we wait on God confidently and quietly. Hebrews 11:1 tells us that faith is the basis of our hope, and later verses illustrate this with a verbal picture gallery of people who had faith during their life struggles. So we want to bring our faith to bear in our health struggles. Stories from the Gospels about people who brought their children and loved ones to Jesus for healing provide us with models for doing the same as we bring our family's needs for healing to Jesus in prayer.

In a single week, three people came to talk to Jake about depression. Clearly this was a health concern for a significant number of people in the Springfield Presbyterian congregation; if three folks had been courageous enough to confess the condition, how many more were struggling in silence? Jake decided that he would devote his next column in the church newsletter to the topic. He did his research first, consulting not only medical resources but also contacting a local pastoral counselor and asking one of the pastoral staff to confirm the biblical material he wanted to include. His goal was to offer people scriptural wisdom as well as practical advice for identifying the signs of depression in themselves and others, and some good strategies for addressing the condition. (See "Sample Church Newsletter Column" at http://www.judson press.com/free_download_book_excerpts.cfm.)

Community Liaison. Many nurses comment to each other, "I am glad I'm a nurse. I would not be able to help my family through the maze of medical care they need if I did not have my nursing background." The average person can be confused by the many changes and options available in the current healthcare network. "Hospitalists" who provide hospitalized patients with care comprise one more group that has recently been added to the network's maze. Coupling this with insurance requirements and the availability of public health programs and services makes finding and receiving care complex. A PN can be a valuable resource to church members who find themselves bewildered by the availability or sometimes inaccessibility of medical-related services and benefits. This role is illustrated by the following account.

One day Nina was pleasantly surprised by a visit from Ernest, the out-of-town son of two older church members. He was hoping she might have some suggestions for helping his parents find a better residence to accommodate their growing needs. "You may know that my parents were missionaries for many years. They have a small retirement pension, but not enough for them to live in any of the local care facilities." He was particularly concerned because his mother was suffering from dementia and needed significant care that his father was struggling to provide.

"Maybe you and I could stop by the local care centers. I don't have any of the flyers left," Nina apologized. "But you'll want to see the facilities for yourself anyway while you're here. We can also stop by the local senior services department. They could do an assessment to determine if one or both of your parents might be eligible for Medicaid or other assistance."

In the meantime, Nina also recommended that Ernest look into the local Meals on Wheels program to relieve his father of grocery and food preparation responsibilities, and she gave him information about a personal medical alert button intended for the elderly to wear at home in case of a fall or other incapacitating incident. If cost for the service was prohibitive, Nina offered to put him in touch with the deacons at the church. "Their benevolence fund should be available for something like that," she assured him.

Volunteer Coordinator. Because a significant part of a PN's ministry is often planning and facilitating health-related events, a common role of the PN is volunteer coordinator. Particularly when an event partners with other organizations or welcomes people from the community (who may be members of other faith communities or neighborhood residents of no church membership), a wide array of volunteers are typically needed. Consider your facility and how it will be used. You may need parking lot attendants; registration table staff; teams for setup and teardown; and greeters or ushers who can welcome participants and provide basic information about restrooms, accessibility, and program locations. Other events may require volunteers with more training or specialized skills, such as people with CPR or first-aid certification to assist in demonstrations, or individuals who can be taught to help with body-mass evaluations or weigh-ins. The example provided here identifies the PN work with health fair volunteers.

In order to sponsor a community health fair, Mary knew that she would need assistants. One thing she did was to put a note on the bulletin board and in the Sunday bulletin telling about the fair and asking for volunteers. She scheduled a basic orientation session for general volunteers, and she planned a second, longer training session for people who would help with record keeping and health assessments. She realized that these assistants would also need instruction on confidentiality of information.

Don't be surprised or discouraged if you have to reach out personally to recruit some volunteers; some people inevitably wait to be asked. Others may need a personal invitation to feel a confidence boost and affirmation of their competency before agreeing to more specialized roles. Be sure to use both public and personal touches not only in recruiting but in thanking your volunteers after the event is over. Make sure each participant knows how vital his or her role was in making the experience a success, and keep track of everyone who participated so that you can include them in any annual appreciation occasion that the church at large may hold. You might also give volunteers the opportunity to provide feedback on the experience so that you can note what worked—and what needs to be changed, added, or omitted in the future.

The background and educational preparation for the PN is quite specific and the key practice guidelines need to be followed. But within the parameters, the role of the PN might be adjusted if a given church has needs unrelated to the roles provided.

Questions

1. Considering the needs of your church, what additional activities and behaviors would you like to add to the PN role?

2. What kinds of health counseling situations have you or a family member had that you would have liked to discuss with a PN?

3. Why do the activities of the parish nurse sometimes change?

4. How would you name the person who works in your church to promote health and integrate faith and health?

Notes

1. Deborah L. Patterson and Mary Slutz, "Faith Community/Parish Nursing: What's in a Name?" *Journal of Christian Nursing* 28, no. 1 (2011): 31–33.

2. Go to IPNRC website at www.parishnurses.org and select Parish Nurse Education Course.

3. L. J. Mayhugh and K. H. Martens, "What's a Parish Nurse to Do?" *Journal of Christian Nursing* 18, no. 3 (2011): 15.

4. Rita P. Wilson, "What Does a Parish Nurse Do?" *Journal of Christian Nursing* 14, no. 1 (1997): 13–15.

5. Granger Westberg, "A Personal Historical Perspective of Whole Person Health and the Congregation," in *Parish Nursing*, ed. Phyllis Ann Solari-Twadell and Mary Ann McDermott (Thousand Oaks, CA: Sage Publications, 1999): 38.

CHAPTER 3

Organization and Accountability in the Church

At the inception of a parish nurse (PN) program in a congregation, it is essential to clarify where the PN fits within the organization of the church administration, the congregation, and the surrounding community.

In most church structures, the pastoral staff, lay leadership (elders or deacons), PN, and healthcare team (or committee) form the center. The PN relates directly to the church leadership. The healthcare team members, through the PN, direct issues of health concerns, such as the purchase of an automatic electronic defibrillator (AED), to the church administrators (secretary, administrative assistant, board of trustees). There should be a reciprocal relationship between members of both groups—the healthcare team and the church administration. In this model the congregation also reciprocally relates to the church administration. The congregation usually connects with the PN and healthcare team at milestone events such as birth, marriage, illness, and death.

On healthcare issues the PN is the natural link connecting professional medicine with the church group that includes people spanning different life stages, socioeconomic levels, and cultural groups. Because the PN is one of the administrative personnel, building space and financial resources can be used for events planned for the church congregation and the larger community.

The church community typically reflects the concerns of persons within the geographical area surrounding the church complex. It becomes a prototype for program plans that might also relate to members outside the congregation. Such programs can be useful as tools for outreach to draw community people into the church. For instance, an annual church-sponsored health fair would include topics of interest throughout the life cycle as well as health prevention aspects related to priority physical problems (obesity, diabetes, etc.), mental health (bullying, loss of relationships, mental abuse and neglect, etc.), and spiritual values (church teaching and beliefs regarding medical decisions, divorce, elderly care, etc.).

Typically a health-related budget is identified annually. The PN, in conjunction with the healthcare team, decides how to allocate funds with respect to program priorities. Costs may include resource speakers and materials. But within the church, a variety of resources also exist. In addition to personnel such as clergy and office staff, the church may have a library and learning resources as well as a communication structure of printed informational bulletins, bulletin boards, and newsletters. Volunteers from the church as well as other church denominational affiliations may be available as helpful resources.

Description of PN Interface with Health Concerns

Health concerns surface in many ways in addition to a formal assessment of needs. According to the organizational pattern, the PN would initiate activities to meet evident health needs or other specific requests. The following examples illustrate how health needs may be brought to the PN's attention.

1. One of the deacons (who happens to be a bacteriologist) tells Jake that frequently after a Sunday service he or his wife will come down with a cold or sinus infection. The deacon has observed that this is common after sitting next to people who were coughing without covering their nose and mouth throughout the morning worship service. Positing a lack of knowledge on the part of some church members about infec-

tious disease, Jake decides to plan a workshop about the spread of organisms, with the deacon-bacteriologist as keynote speaker. In the interim, Jake prepares a bulletin board display for the church lobby, illustrating the cycle of communicable disease transmission.

2. The pastor reports to Dolores that he is concerned about several children from the same family sleeping throughout the worship service. He is used to people dozing off in service occasionally, but when four children between five and ten years of age fall asleep every week, he is concerned. Are the children sleep-deprived, sick, or just bored? Dolores invites the parents to come in for a private health counseling session and asks about the children's apparent need for more sleep. Together, they agree to try an earlier bedtime—and to make use of the children's church service where the kids might be more engaged and better educated in age-appropriate ways. Because Dolores soon observes the issue is relevant beyond this single family, she creates a bulletin insert with advice on ensuring adequate rest and tips for getting good sleep; she will put it in the bulletin in the weeks immediately before and after school opening in the fall.

3. A community request from a public health official asks the church to be the site for a Red Cross blood donation day. The church secretary relays the request to the PN, Nina. Upon securing permission from the pastor, Nina responds to the official by proposing a few possible dates for the event. After settling on the date and time, she helps with organizational details such as reserving the space required, promoting the event in the congregation, and securing church volunteers to assist with the event.

Accountability of the Parish Nurse

In an organizational structure the PN is accountable to the church administration for her or his work performance. Sometimes issues that are acceptable in the nursing/medical professional community may be unacceptable to the church community. An example might be the use of alternative therapies based on Buddhist teachings regarding meditation.

Many other conflicting issues might be identified. A long-standing issue is whether immunizations should be required for children attending public schools. Faith healing might be the approach of some church groups with members who practice this, but these practices may be unacceptable within the professional community for particular illnesses and age groups (the very old and young). Euthanasia and contraception are two other issues that could divide a church community as they often do in the professional community.

In situations where the PN might personally agree with the stance of the health profession, it would be essential that the matter be reviewed with the church administration. The PN would need to support the church position even though it differs from his or her personal and professional view, but it would be helpful for everyone's views to be represented. For example, the question of training and using the automatic electrical defibrillator unit in the church community may inspire controversy. The PN might favor the AED's use if adequate training for ushers and other personnel who would be authorized to use it were provided. However, some in the church might view a situation in which the use of a defibrillator for resuscitation would be interfering with God's chosen "time to die" (Ecclesiastes 3:2, RSV) for the individual.

Structuring the Healthcare Team

Recruitment

Consider questions such as the following when preparing to recruit church members to serve on the healthcare team:

1. Who are the informal leaders within your congregation?
2. Which healthcare professionals are represented in your congregation?

3. What are the informal communication channels that operate in your congregation?

4. What do these representatives and special interest groups identify as priority healthcare needs for the congregation?

5. What are the defining demographic characteristics of your congregation? Consider age and family makeup, employment/retirement statistics, urban/suburban/rural residency, special focus areas (e.g., substance abuse, homelessness, returning veterans), and mission projects or other interests.

Seven or eight people who represent an array of the characteristics of the congregation should be asked to serve on the healthcare committee. Members need to understand that they will be asked for their views and for their help with planning for the health needs of the congregation. Initially this usually requires more frequent meetings, but over time, monthly meetings may suffice. The meetings will be held to review plans, suggest direction, and recruit from or delegate to the committee assistants in conducting some workshops and other healthcare activities.

The PN is usually responsible for initiating plans to recruit people to serve on the committee. Since health professionals would be identified with healthcare, the PN would be wise to call a meeting specifically of the congregational health professionals to apprise them of the activities and role the PN is assuming. This would allow those who might be interested in the new ministry to volunteer to serve on the team. These professionals might then suggest persons who are leaders in key social and other groups to serve on this team.

The PN would review a tentative list of names with designated representatives from the pastoral team and church administration. With approval from this group, the PN would formulate the healthcare team. A subsequent meeting should then be set up to identify the vision and purpose for the committee. The PN would initially serve as facilitator and the team could vote on a chairperson.

Accountability

Members of this committee typically report to the PN with suggestions from their professional groups, the congregation, and the surrounding neighborhood community. Committee members could formally submit issues or may informally identify these in conversation with the PN. The PN in turn would represent the identified issues and concerns to the pastoral team and the church administration.

The PN may selectively present concerns to different administrative groups. For example, a concern with icy parking lots might be brought to the board of trustees or to whatever other group is responsible for maintaining the church and grounds. A concern about directional signage on the church doors (so that in an emergency the ambulance driver and medical technicians might immediately proceed to the door nearest the person needing help) might also go to the trustees. Requests for particular educational content or specific presenters may need to go to the pastoral team, especially if the proposed content involves theologically controversial issues such as euthanasia or do-not-resuscitate orders.

Once the PN role is established in the church at large, more items may be brought to the church administration, to the healthcare committee, or to both groups for review and action. Over time both the administrative members and the PN will develop awareness of key areas that need careful review. For most healthcare issues, the PN and the healthcare team should have the professional knowledge and background to decide when and who should be involved in health program decision-making.

Mary, Newly Inducted PN in Mountain View Church

Mary breathed a sigh of relief after her first meeting with the church administration. That was not so bad, she thought. The church leadership had asked her about her first steps as their PN. That question was easy to answer: she wanted to establish and meet with her healthcare committee. The administrative group had even suggested names for her to contact. She would start there, but she had some other folks in mind as well.

Mary decided that her first task was to draft a letter to Mountain View's church members who had medical training (nurses, EMTs and paramedics, physical therapists, physicians, dentists, etc.), inviting them to a coffee time between the two morning services. She knew that several had not come to the general health professional meeting. She wanted to let them know key details and answer questions they had about the PN role. She also wanted to share details about what she planned to do. She guessed that some of them had heard about this kind of "church" nursing, but they would not have much knowledge of what it actually entailed. She smiled to herself as she realized that she wasn't very sure about what it really involved either.

A couple weeks later, Mary paused to ask the Lord for guidance as she prepared for the first meeting of her healthcare team. She knew most of the people coming and prayed that she could focus their time and energy toward promoting church healthcare. She was prepared with handouts: (1) a detailed description of the PN role, and (2) a sample purpose statement and goals she had obtained from another church's healthcare team (see Appendix A). She hoped the sample would make her team's task easier.

In the hour-long meeting, the team devoted forty-five minutes to brainstorming components of their healthcare team's purpose and goal statement. Mary asked for the working drafts that different members had put together during the discussion, promising to try combining ideas in order to present a second draft at their next meeting two weeks later.

Following the meeting Mary felt invigorated, encouraged by the interest the members showed and the extensive background the various members possessed. She reviewed the membership as she drove home.

Ted: the deacon responsible for health at Mountain View; employed as administrator for a local computer company.

Betty: currently a homemaker with three children under age ten, one of whom was on the autism spectrum; previously a schoolteacher for five years.

Kate: employed at the local geriatric care center; had professional and personal experience as she helped her mother-in-law cope with her father-in-law's degenerative mental illness.

Bill: retired from the Army where he served as a medic; volunteer with fire departments, search and rescue teams, and other organizations dealing with emergencies.

Paula: a registered nurse who worked on an orthopedic floor; an expert in rehabilitation following bone surgery; personal experience in caring for a son who was paralyzed following a head injury.

Eunice: a pharmacist familiar with many drugs that were commonly used; experience in conducting workshops on medication administration issues for professionals and lay people.

Note that among the members of Mary's healthcare team, some people had professional training and expertise in medicine or healthcare areas. Others had personal experience as caregivers or advocates for family members with health concerns. You will benefit from having clinical expertise as well as life experience on your team because the congregation will want assurance of compassion as well as competence in this ministry. And don't forget to seek at least a couple members who will be able and willing to assist with administrative and organizational details!

With a good team for support and collaboration, a PN can feel more confident about approaching the work. A shared sense of purpose and common goals will be invaluable in directing a new parish nursing ministry, and the healthcare team will form a core of volunteers to promote and facilitate programming in the church and community. With such a team's backing, the PN can begin to focus on some of the health needs of the church. The next step? Consider doing a church-wide health assessment, which will be discussed in Chapter 4.

Questions

1. Where would the PN fit into the structural model of your congregation? To whom would the PN report?

2. How might PN accountability be measured in your church organization?

3. How do you envision a healthcare team functioning in your congregation?

4. Consider the demographic characteristics of your congregation. What kind of people should be represented on your church's healthcare committee? Brainstorm a short list of names and solicit other suggestions from your church leadership.

5. In your church setting, which person or group would decide the health focus for the year? Pastor? Church board? Healthcare team? PN?

CHAPTER 4

Church Community Assessment and Planning

A great way for any parish church nurse to begin ministry is to get a good snapshot of the congregation's health-related beliefs, values, and felt needs. What do church members know (or think they know) about physical, mental, and emotional health? How does their faith connect (or fail to connect) to their beliefs about health and its importance to individual and community well-being? What do parishioners themselves say are the most critical health concerns facing them personally or confronting the congregation or community at large? A congregational survey that answers these key questions will be an invaluable tool in ultimately devising a one-year plan for health ministry in your local church.

Survey of Faith Community — Questionnaire

Start by reviewing general healthcare questionnaires in any medical clinic or healthcare facility. Note the various categories covered in the samples, and identify at least five categories to cover in your own assessment tool. (A generic sample that one PN used is included as Appendix B.) You can choose the categories and specific questions that you think would be particularly relevant to your ministry context. For example, Nina serves a congregation in a community with two very different demographics: middle- to upper-class seniors (single, married, and widowed) who had the means to retire with a measure of independence, and Latino families whose extensive family networks included varying socioeconomic levels and documentation status. In contrast, Dolores serves a predominantly African American congregation, with middle-class members who commute to church and a culturally diverse neighborhood with residents who tend to subsist at the poverty line. Dolores may need to identify some health concerns that are shared by parishioners and their neighbors (e.g., type 2 diabetes or sickle cell anemia) as well as concerns that may be deemed more "missions and outreach" than "member education and self-care" (e.g., addiction support groups).

Generally speaking, all church-wide health assessments will need to cover two common categories to start: demographic data and current health status. In other words, concerning the former, a survey should solicit (anonymously) the respondent's gender and age (within a range is fine), as well as other personal data deemed relevant (e.g., race/ethnicity, zip code, marital status, number of children and their ages, frequency of church attendance). Other questions can get at general health status by broad description (e.g., On a scale of 1–5, where 1 is "poor" and 5 is "excellent," how would you rate your physical health? your mental health? your emotional health?) and by typical health concerns (e.g., In the past five years, have you or a member of your household been diagnosed with: a chronic physical condition, a major illness such as cancer, an injury/trauma, an emotional or mental health concern?).

As Jake considered identifying categories for the health assessment for his ministry setting, he settled on the admittedly artificial differentiation of body, mind, and spirit as three of his key areas for evaluation. He knew that the three were inextricably interrelated throughout life—that physical illness took a toll on psycho-emotional health, and that stress or depression often manifested in physical ways, for example. However, he thought that for the purposes of the survey, the distinct categories would be useful. Accordingly, he developed the following list of issues under each of those categories. (What would you add or delete?)

Body	Mind	Spirit
Cardiovascular	Consciousness	Belief and
Gastrointestinal	Understanding	meaning
Skin	Knowledge	Rituals and
Musculoskeletal	Memory	practices
Neurological	Reason	Courage and
Respiratory	Judgment and	growth
	decision-making	Authority and
Genitourinary	Relationships and	guidance
	communication	
Reproductive	Stress	
Eye-Ear-Nose-Throat	Anger	
	Fear and anxiety	
	Mood swings	
	Grief	
	Depression	

Jake decided to organize questions related to the body according to the pattern used in general or family practice medicine. One question for each area would work well. For the category distinguished as "mind," Jake opted against technical jargon in this category, preferring emotional and psychological terms that most church members would understand and identify with.

Jake reviewed his nursing school resources in the area of spiritual care. He recalled that it was a growing area in nursing care over the past decade or so. Based on this review he decided on four subcategories, with short-answer questions for two and objective responses for two:[1]

> (1) **Belief and meaning:** such as understanding God's providence, especially related to human suffering or sin.

Q: What gives meaning and purpose to your life?

(2) **Rituals and practices:** such as Communion, baptism, prayer, and worship.

Q: What are the religious or faith-based rituals that provide structure for your everyday life?

(3) **Courage and growth:** such as a sense of future hope and the ability to discover meaning in life's daily changes.

Q: How courageous or hopeful are you?

_____ Very

_____ Somewhat

_____ Not at all

(4) **Authority and guidance:** such as how we develop or affirm personal perspectives on health, illness, or injury.

Q: Where do you find authority for your life?

_____ Scripture

_____ Religious beliefs and teachings

_____ Friends and family

_____ Other _____

Another area to explore in a congregational health assessment would be the educational needs of the congregation, specifically related to physical and mental health. These needs may be uncovered through observation or anecdotes as the PN begins ministry in the local church or community. For example, Mary had a counseling session with a member newly diagnosed with adult-onset diabetes. The parishioner was overwhelmed with the diagnosis and all the information provided by the doctor—and Mary knew that she needed to provide a kind of cheat sheet to ease the learning curve for the member and the member's family. Similarly, Nina was delighted to be introduced to the hearing impaired family member of another parishioner, and Nina knew that the congregation would need a crash course in conversational sign language and the unique needs of the deaf and hearing impaired in order to make this visitor truly welcome. Be sure to include questions on your survey that allow church members to identify their own priority learning needs, such as the following:

- What health concern do you need to know more about NOW?
- What health concern would you like to know more about in the FUTURE?
- Where do you usually go for information about health concerns? (Rank your top three sources below.)
  - My personal physician
  - The Internet (WebMD.com, Wikipedia, Ask.com)
  - The local library
  - Popular media (*Dr. Oz*, newspaper or magazine articles)
  - A friend or relative with medical experience
  - A friend or relative with similar concerns
  - Parish/church nurse
  - Other _____

Finally, don't neglect to include questions that will help you create a strategy for addressing immediate felt needs and match congregational resources with those needs. What do church members identify as their greatest health-related need? Are there people or ministries in the church that are already equipped to help meet that need? (See the sample questionnaire in Appendix B—especially the section on questions relating to Needs and Help Available on page 137.)

For example, Nina's church assessment revealed a number of young parents who desperately needed childcare so that they could attend job interviews and ESL classes—and also a lot of healthy retirees who desperately missed having grandchildren close by to nurture and spoil! And Mary discovered that many of her seniors were in failing health and requiring transportation to their many medical appointments; she contacted the coordinator of the church's existing transportation ministry to ask if drivers might be available during the week for such trips. Sure enough, the answer was yes! Dolores learned that several members of her congregation were anxious about teenagers at home with little to occupy them and few summer jobs available in the community—while other parishioners were seeking assistance with occasional childcare, errands, or routine chores around house and yard. What a great way to encourage relationships among individuals and across generations, while simultaneously meeting real needs in the church family.

Questionnaire Review and Administration

After you have drafted the survey tool, be sure to share it with your healthcare team for their feedback. It's a great idea to have them "beta test" the survey by completing it themselves. See how long it takes and if there are any challenges with the form or technology. If appropriate, share the tool with your pastoral staff or church governing board as well. Your beta testers will probably have helpful suggestions, and they or the church leadership may also have strong recommendations (or requirements) for how the survey should be distributed (e.g., mailed via postal service, sent through electronic communication, handed out in person at an event).

If your congregation is generally computer-savvy and technologically connected, consider using an online survey tool such as SurveyMonkey or Google Forms for easy tallying of responses. You can send out a hyperlink to the survey via e-mail or by posting it in the church bulletin. Be sure to have some hard copies available for the people who don't have access to or familiarity with such online tools. You can always integrate those responses manually. If you have a church comprised predominantly of "old school" members, however, stick with a paper-and-pencil questionnaire and identify at least two occasions when surveys can be distributed and collected in the same day or hour to maximize responses.

Regardless of whether you choose an electronic or paper format, keep the survey short and sweet—limited in length and complexity so that parishioners can and will complete it in roughly ten minutes. A quarterly church business meeting might be a good forum for distribution, instruction, and collection of hard-copy surveys, with follow-up opportunities at a well-attended midweek Bible study or adult Sunday school class. Additional questionnaires can always be made available for people to pick up after Sunday worship service and dropped off at the church office or in a box created for that purpose in the church lobby.

Analyzing Questionnaire Data

As noted above, an online survey tool will automatically tally and analyze responses to your questionnaire. If your church is "old school," however, your analysis will need to be "old school" too! Demographic data are usually straightforward to compile and analyze. Create a spreadsheet or similar tool for tallying the number of male/female responses, as well as the breakdown in other categories. With respect to general health status, the ease of compiling the data will depend on the number of questions and the complexity of solicited responses. But be sure to identify what percentage of the church identified their overall status as "good" versus "poor," and highlight specific areas commonly flagged as "poor," whether in specific age groups or across all ages (e.g., exercise routine, stress management).

Under "sources of health information," note which source is most popular/common and which is least used. If "parish/church nurse" is low in the rankings, then you know you need to do some self-promotion of the ministry—but you may also need to bring in outside professionals whose expertise and knowledge is more universally acknowledged and respected. Many congregations have a learning curve when it comes to the parish nurse ministry itself. Perhaps an informational session about what the PN will do in the congregation would be good. Some attendees might give suggestions for learning interests at this session. It may take time before church members learn to recognize and value their PN as a source of invaluable information and service.

For the questions related to parishioner-identified learning needs, consider grouping the responses by age, in ten- to twenty-year increments. Assuming you had few to no respondents in the 0–19 age bracket, begin with 20–29 (ten years) or 40–59 (twenty years). Ideally, you will have asked respondents to rank the learning areas. Depending on how many you asked them to rank (top two, top five, etc.), you may choose to analyze only the primary and secondary areas (first and second choices). Keep the others on file somewhere. But these primary and secondary responses may form the basis for your one-year health ministry plan. (See Appendix C for a sample spreadsheet with primary and secondary learning priorities grouped by ten-year age ranges.)

Jake discovered that all ages identified exercise as a primary need; he made a particular note of that area for its intergenerational program potential. Similarly stress management was a concern identified by all ages except the 70+ group, so he flagged that as a priority for early in his one-year plan.

Nina was confused at first when she saw the diversity of needs expressed by her 60–69 age group. But then she considered her demographics. Many of her 60-somethings were still employed in their fields or were recent retirees who were active and independent, physically as well as financially. Others were struggling with chronic health concerns or devastating illness. Some were raising grandchildren or supporting other family members in some kind of life transition.

When Dolores saw the tabulated responses under spiritual needs, she decided to share the information with the pastor. Some identified specific areas where they wanted more education, such as prayer and spiritual maturity. Many noted that their faith gave meaning and purpose to their lives, but more than half indicated they needed other people to guide them during difficult times. The pastor was glad to have the data: "These areas will provide good topics for our small group ministry in the coming year," Rev. Carter told Dolores with gratitude.

Don't be overwhelmed by the information you glean from the assessment. Don't feel responsible for meeting all the needs identified!

Like Dolores and Mary in the preceding illustrations, feel free to refer certain information to other experts in the church—the pastor, a pastoral counseling service, even the transportation ministry! And remember that your healthcare committee is there, along with the church staff, to support and advise. Don't hesitate to call in resource people from the congregation or community to contribute from their area of expertise.

Administering the questionnaires and then analyzing the results will take time, even if you do take advantage of technology. But the time spent on assessment will be well worth the effort. The information you compile will be invaluable as you prepare to plan your ministry in the coming months. Equipped with such rich, voluntary data, you can create programs and services that truly meet the expressed needs of your church family.

Developing a Plan for Year One

After doing a church-wide assessment and analyzing the responses, the parish church nurse should be equipped to map out a one-year ministry plan for maximum impact on church and community. That doesn't mean the task will be simple or easy! But you should have some handles for identifying priority health concerns and for structuring programs suited to the congregation.

Begin with the expressed needs of the survey respondents. These become the anchors for the one-year plan. Depending upon the number and variety of priority learning areas identified by the congregation, you might choose four of them as your quarterly themes (e.g., nutrition, exercise, stress management, aging), or you might be able to highlight a different issue each month or bimonthly. Be cautious about planning too much in any given year, especially with a new ministry. Appendix D provides a sample plan for one year.

Jake was new to the role of PN, and the health ministry was only a year or two "older" than his position. So, when he looked at the calendar for the next twelve months, Jake decided that it would be sufficiently ambitious for him to plan just two major health-related events this year. He would have a steep learning curve in the planning process, and he knew that church members would need time to discover the value and transformational potential of the health ministry—not only for them as individuals, but also for the congregation as a whole and its relationship with the community. After consulting with his healthcare team, Jake settled on an educational workshop on stress management to kick off the year and a men's health fair in the fall, which would coincide nicely with Prostate Cancer Awareness Month in September.

Such national awareness months also ensure that a PN has plenty of great promotional materials and supporting educational resources available to support a local church focus. An Internet search of "national awareness months" should yield an impressive list. Don't attempt to highlight all of them each year! But you might want to keep track of the ones you do emphasize this year so that you can plan accordingly in years to come. Some emphases will be so successful that church members will clamor for a repeat annually (e.g., participation in the local 5K run to raise funds and awareness for breast cancer); others will make good reprises every two or three years (e.g., intergenerational fun day for families of children with autism). And some themes or issues may be vital one year (e.g., depression, after a church member commits suicide) and supplanted by another congregational concern another year (e.g., adoption and foster care when a new family joins the church).

In planning, also be strategic about a diversity of approaches to education, information, and participation. Offer church members a variety of options for engagement—not only as volunteers but as attendees. The PN and healthcare team aren't the only ones who will burn out from too many major activities. The congregation is busy and often overcommitted as well. Think about low-level engagement opportunities, such as a regular PN column in the church newsletter or informational inserts in the Sunday bulletin. Consider mid-level options as well, such as weekly exercise classes, weight loss support groups, or a rotating team of volunteers for monthly visitation of members who are homebound or hospitalized. Then decide on just a couple high-level activities, perhaps one that involves joining with a community effort (e.g., an awareness fundraiser) and one that invites the community in (e.g., an educational workshop or health fair).

Dolores had already noted the high priority her congregation had placed on learning about exercise. And with weight loss and improved physical health being a popular New Year's resolution theme for many, why not make exercise her first-quarter theme? She could introduce the emphasis and outline her schedule for the coming months in her PN column in the January newsletter. For February, she could put together key facts and distribute them as a bulletin insert and post other information on the health bulletin board. Then in March she could get a physical fitness expert, whether from the congregation or the local fitness club, to present a demonstration workshop with exercises for all ages, including "senior-cise" that would focus on gentle stretching. This workshop might be held in the church's fellowship hall so participants could divide into groups and actually practice an exercise routine.

Mary had been serving her church as PN for several years, and the health ministry was thriving. After a slow start, people really seemed to have caught the vision (much healthier than catching a cold!) and actually called or e-mailed her to ask, "What's next?" With strong volunteer support, Mary felt that she could be more ambitious in her plan for the coming year. And after reviewing the plans from previous years, with notes about which events and themes had been most popular and received the best feedback, she prepared a chart for her healthcare committee and the church leadership. Eventually, she would make the calendar available to the congregation, perhaps on the church website or as a bulletin insert, so everyone could quickly review the one-year plan. She structured the chart with a column for the month, the health focus, potential resource person, and learning activities related to the focus area. (See Appendix D for Mary's one-year planning chart.)

Give yourself time to put together the one-year plan. Depending on your ministry structure and accountability framework, you will likely need to submit it for approval, if only with the church secretary or whatever committee or staff person keeps the church-wide planning calendar. Such a process will require additional time if the plan needs to be submitted to a board or the pastor for input and approval. Even the fairly autonomous PN will benefit from running the plan by his or her healthcare committee. As Proverbs 11:14 says, there is wisdom in a multitude of advisors!

Finally, keep in mind that while details regarding resource people and activities are great, you will need to stay flexible and your calendar will benefit from having some fluidity to it. Even the best plans will be subject to change and revision, whether because of church feedback about dates, or postponements because of weather, or last-minute cancellations by your guest presenter. As long as you communicate clearly and promptly about changes, both to church leadership and to the congregation and community, your program will survive tweaks and revisions with good grace.

Questions

1. How could a health assessment of your congregation be used?

2. In what ways could a survey of learning needs be informative in your PN work?

3. Do you think that needs identified by the church members should take priority over those the PN might choose to focus on? Why or why not?

4. In preparing a one-year plan, how might you balance professionally identified needs (e.g., obesity or heart health) with competing congregational priorities?

5. Why might you like to consider your one-year plan a work-in-progress?

6. In your congregation, who will be involved in reviewing and approving the PN's one-year plan? Pastor, church board, healthcare team, or PN? Why?

Notes

1. For an excellent description of spiritual care, see Judith Allen Shelly's description in *Spiritual Care* (Downers Grove, IL: InterVarsity Press, 2000), 38. You'll find great open-ended assessment questions in Carol J. Farran, George Fitchett, Julia D. Quiring-Emblen, and J. Russell Burck, "Development of a Model for Spiritual Assessment and Intervention," *Institutes of Religion and Health* 28, no. 3 (1989): 185–194. The four categories Jake preferred are in Julia D. Quiring-Emblen and Barbara Pesut, "Strengthening Transcendent Meaning," *Journal of Holistic Nursing* 19, no. 1 (2001): 42–56.

CHAPTER 5

The Parish Nurse Toolbox

Nurses work with a number of pieces of equipment, although they usually don't carry them in a little black bag like doctors do. But working as a PN might require a "toolbox" of sorts, differing from the old medical bag and the carpenter's toolbox. An inventory of the tangible and intangible tools that need to be included might clarify what these are and how they are used. Such a list follows, along with examples of how they assist the PN.

Accessibility

Because church members need to have easy ways to contact their PN whenever needs arise, personal accessibility is a vital aspect of PN ministry. Hours of work should be clearly posted and communicated to all parishioners, but like a pastor, the PN may expect emergencies outside of posted hours. Responding to such crises may require the PN to exercise a measure of wisdom and discretion, both for self-care and for ministry effectiveness. This is particularly critical for the volunteer or part-time PN.

Telephone

An invaluable, tangible tool for the PN is a cell phone dedicated to ministry work. Prompt retrieval of calls is essential with respect to healthcare concerns. When calls come in outside of posted work hours, the voice-mail response should note: "If this is a medical emergency, please hang up and call 9-1-1 immediately. Then if you would like, call back and leave a message so that I can follow up with you as soon as possible."

PNs need to keep a log of their calls for future reference and review. According to Mary's phone call notebook, she logged seventy-five in-coming calls in her first month. (Jake logged roughly the same number of calls—and an equal number of text messages, mostly from the young adult members of the 800-member congregation he served. In contrast, Nina and Dolores, who served smaller congregations, logged twenty-five to thirty calls in an average month.)

Most of the time Mary found people honored her work hours and called her only on the days she had office hours (three days a week). When callers received the message that she was out of the office, most left a voicemail. So far, she has received only one call on her home number, and that was from a church member whose spouse was having chest pains and didn't know whether to call 9-1-1. Understanding the woman's anxiety and knowing the couple well, Mary offered to make the emergency call on their behalf and directed first responders to their home address.

E-mail

E-mails are often used by PNs to confirm meetings or appointments, to coordinate details about upcoming events, or to suggest future programs. E-mail is also the recommended form of communication for contacting professional groups and outside experts who can provide information about some aspect of nursing care.

PNs may find that certain members of the congregation prefer e-mail for personal communication about health and other concerns. One lovely lady had written simply to tell Dolores that she was praying for her, while Jake regularly corresponded with a group of church members who were supporting one another in a new weight loss effort. While Mary found that she had received more than 150 e-mails in her first month, Nina averaged 80 to 90 messages, which included some program organizational calls.

Office Visits

Office Hours. Office hours need to be clearly posted and communicated to the congregation. Depending on the setting, some walk-in time before or after regular church events may be helpful. Some walk-ins may be neighborhood residents who have questions about recurring symptoms or a new diagnosis. Others may be parishioners who come to the church for another meeting but stop in to weigh themselves on the PN's office scale or to ask for a quick blood pressure check. In reviewing her log, Dolores noted that in the twelve hours she worked each week (four hours a day, three days a week), she averaged three appointments a day and one walk-in per week. The walk-ins tended to be most frequent before and after midweek Bible study or choir rehearsals.

Office Appointments. While walk-in hours are a key aspect of parish nurse ministry, scheduled appointments are also beneficial to PNs and parishioners alike. Parishioners will appreciate the convenience of timely attention and a discrete block of time reserved for them and their concerns. PNs will value the potential for advance notice about particular questions or concerns so that they can prepare in advance of the appointment.

Jake was quick to offer his older members an appointment so that they weren't subject to long waits during his walk-in hours. When another parishioner scheduled an appointment to talk about his daughter's diagnosis of autism, Jake was grateful to have time to gather educational materials and community resources in advance.

Office Space. If at all possible, the PN's office should be located near an external door of the church building. Such a location will greatly enhance accessibility because people don't like to hunt for offices. With respect to mobility, consider factors such as steps and distance from the nearest accessible entrance. Privacy poses another concern for a PN ministry. Consider how to create a comfortable and discreet space where people who arrive early for their appointment might sit and wait.

Office furniture arrangement is also important. If possible, the office space should include a small round table so both the PN and parishioner can sit at the table. If space does not allow for this, the PN's desk should be arranged so that the nurse can sit beside the person. When the PN's desk sits between the nurse and parishioner, the physical barrier may create an obstacle to open dialogue. If space permits, keep an extra chair in the office to prevent the awkwardness or inconvenience of finding additional seating should two individuals come to the appointment.

Finally, consider matters of physical comfort. Can you provide access to coffee, hot tea, or cold water? Many people feel more at ease when they have a cup in hand, while others who arrive with cold symptoms or old-fashioned nerves will be grateful for something to wet their whistle. And in light of the PN's health ministry, what about having a supply of facial tissues and hand sanitizer? Don't forget clear directions for finding the restrooms—ideally posted in the office, but also memorized for the simplest possible communication.

Presence

Perhaps the personal presence of the nurse is most clearly identified when the PN visits people in the home or hospital setting. Such visits have an element of spiritual care, much as a pastor's visit would, but the nurse will also ask or field questions that help identify key concerns a parishioner needs to ask a healthcare provider. Also, a nurse's initial observation of a person who is dealing with illness or surgery provides a baseline to identify positive or negative changes on subsequent visits.

The ministry of presence is also powerful on any given Sunday before or after worship service. The weekly time for worship and fellowship provides the PN with opportunities to visit with people in a casual and social environment. Such encounters provide a personal connection between parishioners and the PN so that church members might later feel free to approach the PN with questions about health concerns. If an individual raises such concerns in or around the worship service, the PN can then offer to schedule an office appointment, which allows for privacy and the comfort of chairs and table to deal more extensively with symptoms and other health issues.

Assessment

Congregational Assessment

An initial congregational assessment, as described in Chapter 4, provides the PN with a lot of grouped assessment data that reveal information about the church community. However, it will be helpful to follow up on that initial large-scale evaluation of needs and interests with a more detailed assessment of selected groups—for example, by following up with a specific demographic or with individuals who attended a recent health-focused program or event. Such targeted evaluations provide key details about specific needs and allow the PN to update the congregational profile for ongoing educational needs and other program activities.

For example, four weeks after a workshop on exercise and stress, Mary distributed an abbreviated questionnaire to those who had participated, asking them to respond to questions about changes in exercise habits and things they were implementing to deal with their stress. Upon reviewing responses, Mary found that respondents were struggling with modifying their schedules to incorporate an exercise routine. Those who expressed benefit from the increased exercise identified reduction of muscle tension. Several asked about when to use special stress reduction techniques such as deep breathing. This information allowed Mary to plan a follow-up session to discuss what people did to incorporate daily exercise, and to get an expert to demonstrate and further help people practice the use of stress reduction techniques.

Personal Interactions

PNs should have ample opportunity to develop their interpersonal assessment skills—skills that need no survey or questionnaire to evaluate individuals' concerns or interests. In every encounter with people, take the opportunity to observe them for physical symptoms such as shortness of breath, facial flushing, or blue-tinged fingernails. Simply by talking to someone, the PN can identify whether the individual is confused or using an unusual speech pattern. You can also observe a person's posture and gait and notice whether someone grimaces in pain with particular movements.

Nina found that the church social hour was a helpful time to screen for major concerns. One Sunday morning Nina noticed that Maria was walking peculiarly and suggested that Maria check with her doctor, who referred Maria to a neurologist, who diagnosed multiple sclerosis. During another social time Nina noticed Juan slurring his words more noticeably than usual. She suggested that he check with his doctor, who diagnosed a mild stroke and initiated treatment.

Church Members as Case-Finders

PNs will often find partners among other church members to aid their congregational assessments. People with no special training will frequently observe changes in friends and fellow committee members or Bible study attendees. PNs who have an open-door policy may get valuable tips from church members who come to their office to share particular observations and concerns about changes in behavior, response, or physical condition. In such cases, the PN should be careful about confidentiality. PNs are professionally committed to honor the Health Insurance Portability and Accountability Act (HIPAA), which obligates all healthcare workers to respect privacy relating to medical concerns. Even if others in the church are aware of an individual's health problem, it is not the place of the PN to share information that was imparted in confidence and professional privacy.

Whenever someone mentioned a concern to her, Dolores always expressed her appreciation of the referring person's intervention. However, Dolores was also clear that she would follow up with the affected individual personally—and she was scrupulous about sharing no additional information with the referring church member. If that concerned individual asked, the PN simply offered assurances that the matter was being addressed.

When a friend or family member was kind enough to provide transportation or companionship to an appointment, Jake was warm in his gratitude—and firm in his request for the concerned chauffer to wait in another room so that Jake could talk privately with his patient.

Blood Pressure Screenings

Like the stethoscope, a blood pressure cuff is a tangible tool the PN uses to identify symptoms of illness. However, the dialogue while assessing the person's blood pressure affords a great opportunity to learn even more health-related information. People often reveal their educational needs when they explain why they skipped a medication. Often they have mistaken assumptions about side effects—including supposed side effects that may really be symptoms of other health concerns. Other folks will point to their morning coffee, rather than its lack of accompanying nutritional intake, as the reason for an elevated blood pressure reading. Others provide a window into family relationships and stress levels when they confess to forgetting their recent doses because of a turbulent week at home with houseguests or special office problems. The PN can use these conversations to explain the need for consistent daily schedules when taking medication, and the attentive PN will also make mental—and later, paper—notes regarding other issues that come up and need to be included in educational seminars and discussions.

For example, Mary was amazed that people either did not know, or conveniently forgot about, the effects of elevated blood pressure readings. And based on the frequency of people blaming their blood pressure medications for other symptoms, Mary opted to create a bulletin insert on distinguishing stroke from cardiac symptoms.

For Dolores's regular patients, she made a log so that she could periodically give each person a graph of their weekly blood pressure readings. She distributed the graphs at six-week intervals, placing each graph in a sealed envelope with the patient's name on it and dropping it in the person's church mailbox. However, whenever she found a sharp elevation in a person's reading from one week to the next, she called the person directly and suggested an immediate appointment with a healthcare provider.

Planning

Initially planning does not seem like a tangible tool, but like the "presence" tool, the PN must plan carefully so that findings can be further clarified and treated if necessary. The plan for what to do about any given assessed finding must be put in place so that any requisite care can be provided.

Healthcare Committee

The PN's healthcare committee is typically designated as one of the key planning groups. A well-selected team will bring a variety of informed perspectives to the planning process, and the PN will benefit from having a larger group to consult with on specific issues and unforeseen circumstances.

Jake was incredibly grateful for his healthcare committee. He felt comfortable calling any member for advice on areas with which they were familiar. He certainly had their support in putting together a church assessment survey. They had given him good suggestions about questions to add and how to modify other items. And they had even completed the questionnaire themselves and so became his pilot test group.

Special Interest Groups

Another source for planning comes from parishioner comments and requests. For example, Mrs. Alvarez told Nina that she was a diabetic, and she would welcome the opportunity to meet with others who had diabetes as well. From similar discussions with others, Nina identified an immediate need for two interest groups: one for diabetes maintenance, and another for obesity/weight loss. Nina found that planning small group meetings was a useful "tool" in setting up these two special interest groups to get people with similar concerns together.

Initially Nina wanted to facilitate each of these groups, but she also needed to be sure that she did not overextend her own time. So she, along with members of each of the groups, identified a person to facilitate for each group, individuals who would organize and initiate meetings and propose topics of discussion. Nina wanted to see if these groups would grow without needing her involvement at every meeting.

Pastoral Staff

A PN will soon discover the value of having the support of the pastor and church staff. A senior pastor is in a position to endorse the ministry of the PN and to affirm the PN's efforts to integrate faith and health at the church. Not only will a pastor be able to establish a theological foundation for the church's participation in a healing ministry that is modeled after Christ's own work on earth, but the pastor and church staff will also be influential in facilitating church-wide planning around health-related ministry events.

Mary knew that she could go to the pastoral staff and the leadership group at any time for planning assistance. She was grateful that the deacon board had told her to contact them when she encountered financial needs that related to healthcare. The deacons' fund would be a resource she could count on for help. And she knew that when people had questions about their faith and issues of medical ethics, Pastor Bill was always available to her and to the parishioners with sound biblical counsel and a gracious response.

Ushers

Ushers can assist in planning for needs that arise during church services. For example, they can assist with planning for parishioner emergencies such as falling in a hallway, suffering a seizure during service, and even evacuating in case of fire or other emergency. When ushers observe unusual occurrences, they have to make judgments and plan how to handle emergencies. They need to decide whom to notify, such as the pastor, a physician attending the service, the PN, or a family member, and then assist with obtaining requisite help if needed.

On her second Sunday as a PN, Dolores was introduced to the need for equipping ushers to support in case of medical emergencies. One of the older parishioners apparently fainted during worship service. The ushers quickly called their new PN to help, and while Dolores checked the parishioner, she asked the ushers to call 9-1-1. For some reason they could not decide who was to do this and valuable time was lost before the call was made.

The next day, Dolores called the head usher and asked about setting up guidelines for medical emergencies during a church service. He was eager to talk with her and suggested that she attend the next meeting of the ushers so they could talk about developing a plan. (See Appendix E for an Emergency Plan similar to what Dolores and the ushers finally put into place.)

Program Development (Intervention)

Program development in the context of a parish nurse ministry assumes a level of intervention in the health and wellness of church members. Such intervention might take the form of educational workshops, health screenings, or support groups, but the overarching goal is to intervene for the improved health of individual church members.

With a new program in mind, a PN will need to identify a strategy for developing and implementing the idea. Here are some key questions to consider and answer:

1. How can you communicate the idea and promote the program to the congregation?

2. How will you get people involved in the new program? Will individuals be included automatically, based on current age or health? Or will you invite people to register or sign up?

3. What is the stated purpose of the new program? How often will it function—daily, weekly, monthly, or only "as needed"?

4. Who else should be involved in the planning and implementation of the program? What role might other church staff members have in its initial launch or on an ongoing basis?

Program development is another initially intangible PN tool. As interests, needs, concerns, and problems arise for parishioners, programs offer a way to meet the needs or to intervene to decrease the toll they take.

Educational Programs

Much of parish nurse ministry involves education, or sharing information about health issues and concerns—from nutrition and weight management to addiction and recovery, to adolescence and aging, to disease prevention and treatment. Educational programs might be as simple as a health ministry column in the weekly bulletin or monthly church newsletter; it may be as complex and multifaceted as an annual health fair with guest speakers and specialized workshops.

Nina became aware of a critical need for education in her congregation when an unimmunized eight-year-old who attended Sunday school was diagnosed with measles. As soon as she heard about the diagnosis, Nina contacted the public health department about the need to immunize the adults and children who had had contact with the infected child. The county medical director responded promptly to attend an emergency meeting with Nina and the healthcare committee to determine a course of action. Beyond the immediate treatment of those who had been exposed to the disease, Nina also worked with the county and the healthcare committee to develop a long-term program to educate the congregation about common infectious diseases and the imperative for timely immunizations, especially for children and high-risk adults. The plan included a series of bulletin inserts about specific diseases, a workshop about free immunization clinics and patients' rights, and a panel discussion with Nina and other healthcare providers about the pros and cons of immunizations.

Special Focus Programs

In addition to prevention and treatment education, an attentive PN will soon begin to identify patterns in the expressed needs of church members. In the church Nina served, which included a significant percentage of newly arrived immigrants, one such need was access to free healthcare, especially for children and seniors. For Dolores, a recurring concern seemed to be increasing diagnoses of type 2 diabetes.

It took a couple months before Jake identified a pattern in his setting, because the concern was largely unspoken. But as he looked over his phone logs, Jake noticed a disproportionate number of calls from older parishioners. Although aging typically is accompanied by escalating health concerns, many of these parishioners had only minor complaints—but they called multiple times a month, and sometimes multiple times a week. Of those frequent callers, most were over the age of seventy and lived alone. In the next week or so, Jake listened carefully to these seniors and noted that many of them demonstrated evidence of feeling lonely. He also realized that such elders who lived independently were a vulnerable population, at risk for falls and other sudden health emergencies with no live-in companions to help them. If they weren't calling him, how would he know they were OK? After consulting with his healthcare committee, Jake devised a telephone chain program for seniors. He solicited input from representative seniors and used the church's existing prayer chain model to organize a new chain for shut-in, disabled, and elderly people.

Originally, the purpose of the telephone chain was to confirm the well-being of each person who was called. But Jake soon heard from the participants that the chain had become a lifeline in other ways, fostering new friendships and easing the loneliness that plagued so many of the largely homebound parishioners. (See "Good Morning Call Line" at http://www.judsonpress .com/free_download_book_ excerpts.cfm.)

Evaluation Strategies

Evaluation strategies are a vital "tool," though initially they seem intangible when they are informal, taking the form of anecdotal feedback or other casual verbal communication. Evaluations become more tangible when formalized, such as asking parishioners to complete a short feedback survey after a workshop or doing exit interviews with participants following a screening. Effective evaluation strategies can empower a PN and healthcare committee to implement specific changes in response to people's feedback.

Informal Strategies

Dolores had developed a routine when she met one-on-one with parishioners. She never let someone leave without posing at least one simple question to solicit some measure of input or feedback on the parish nurse ministry as a whole. She would ask someone who regularly participated in blood pressure screenings, "How did you feel about the new process I introduced last Sunday?" She would ask someone who had attended a recent support group, "What did you think about the guest speaker last month?" She would ask a teen, "Do you think your friends at school or in youth group would be interested in training together for a half marathon?" And she would ask a parent of school-aged children, "What kind of health issues do you think are the biggest concern for young parents today?"

Some people shrugged or answered noncommittally, but Dolores had also gotten some great feedback and helpful ideas from her informal polling efforts. Some comments could be implemented immediately; others she filed away for future reference. But in all cases, she valued additional information about the health preferences of individuals in the congregation.

Formal Strategies

More formal evaluation strategies are those that a PN can develop in consultation with the healthcare committee. You don't want to overwhelm parishioners with requests for feedback. Most people will get weary of taking surveys after each event. But selective polling of representative participants or individuals in a target population (based on age, diagnosis, season of life, etc.) can be useful in assessing the success of a specific program or the ongoing effectiveness of the parish nurse ministry overall. (See Appendix F for a sample program evaluation form.)

Professional Knowledge and Background

As a professional healthcare worker, the parish nurse's education and practical experience provide effective tools for observation and making educated judgments about a person's symptoms, appearance, behavior, or verbal expression. Nurses with training usually can make important judgments within their areas of background preparation. For example, most nurses could look at a person's back and identify scoliosis (S-curvature of the spine); such observation would lead to a referral, first to a primary care physician and perhaps ultimately to an orthopedic surgeon. A nurse with experience in a school setting might recognize characteristics that would suggest that a child is on the autism spectrum, while someone with experience in assisted living facilities will readily identify symptoms of early-onset Alzheimer's. Having a parish nurse who is not only clinically trained but also pursuing ongoing professional development and continuing education will be invaluable to a congregation.

Formal Education

Formal education begins with a degree in nursing from an accredited school. Whether the parish nurse is an RN or LPN/LVN, that credential speaks to his or her preparation for the role. Formal education is also gained on the job as a nurse pursues a particular specialty or field of practice. And continuing education opportunities, in healthcare and other areas of ministry, will foster a lifetime learning model that keeps the PN up-to-date on current research and new trends in healthcare.

Mary knew that her own professional knowledge provided her a helpful foundation as she provided care as a PN. Her bachelor's degree in nursing had provided her with knowledge and experience caring for individual patients and in working with groups with more advanced healthcare needs—information that the community as a whole needed for managing chronic illnesses such as diabetes. Her work in a community health position gave her background in attempting to meet needs that people experienced in a community context.

Dolores valued the experience she had gained each day working in a small general hospital. She had developed good clinical and management skills that ultimately earned her a promotion to clinical supervisor. She had worked with both maternal and child health programs as well as with geriatric populations. She was responsible for identifying needs for these population groups and then setting up programs to meet the needs. This experience helped her immensely in her PN role.

Proud of his newly earned nursing degree, Jake realized that he didn't have any biblically based education. He decided that when it was feasible, he would enroll in some courses at the nearby seminary. He thought that courses in church history and health and healing in the Bible might be useful in his PN role. He wanted to be able to speak the same language as the pastoral team and also become more familiar with various theological questions and concerns so that he could interpret these issues to the parishioners who sought his advice and care.

Life Experiences

As with members of the healthcare committee, the life experiences of a parish nurse will supplement formal education and enrich ministry with parishioners. Life experience not only offers familiarity with common concerns, but also offers practical knowledge of needed resources. And don't overlook the value of compassion, which is deepened when the PN can honestly say, "I know how you feel."

Nina was grateful for her own life experiences that enabled her to understand families' problems more personally and to help them deal with those issues. Nina's aunt had been homebound for years as a result of residual paralysis from polio, and Nina had helped her *tia* with housekeeping chores and other basic needs. Similarly, Nina's cousin had been ill with cancer for a number of years, and Nina had helped the family provide some care. Those experiences made Nina an empathetic listener and an advocate for caregivers as well as their patients.

Mary had two children, and she had been a nurse for them through all the childhood communicable diseases and teenage struggles. Her husband constantly struggled with weight, and so she knew firsthand what this struggle entailed for the family. She found that those experiences equipped her to respond with humor and sympathy to parents and spouses who worried about supporting their families in making healthy choices.

Dolores was a cancer survivor herself. That experience added practical knowledge, emotional empathy, and spiritual wisdom to her PN toolbox. She could sense the fear in a newly diagnosed parishioner, the exhaustion in a patient going through chemo, and the despair in a person who had just heard the treatment wasn't successful. She also had some creative ideas for rallying hope, restoring peace, and seeking support—ideas that she had implemented in her own journey and that she could testify really worked.

Resources

Resources become a requisite tool for every professional. With many complex needs presenting, no given professional can know all things every person needs.

Local and National
A parish nurse will receive innumerable notifications via e-mail, social media, and regular mail announcing local blood drives, awareness weeks/months, health drives, advocacy runs, regional workshops and training events, and more. Consider creating a bulletin board or webpage for posting such notices, and let the congregation know where to look for the information.

Additionally, a PN will want to compile a list of national and local organizations that can be valuable resources for information, education, and training. This list might be posted publicly or it might be kept in a binder or directory in the PN office, where it is easily accessible when the need arises. The following is a chart of national organizations, to which you can add as appropriate.

Figure 1 / Sample List of Resources
*Local chapters listed online or in phone book

Name	Address	Type of Assistance
Alzheimer's Association	225 N Michigan Ave Suite 1700 Chicago, IL 60601 (800) 272-3900 (toll-free) www.alz.org	Provides information and support services to people and families with AD; supports research
American Association of Homes and Services for the Aging	2519 Connecticut Avenue NW Washington, DC 20008 (202) 783-2242 www.aahsa.org	Source of information on long-term care
American Association of Retired Persons	601 E Street NW Washington, DC 20049 (202) 434-2277 (800) 424-3410 (toll-free) www.aarp.org/drive	Provides information for multiple problems related to aging, e.g., driving class
American Diabetes Association	701 N Beauregard Street Alexandria, VA 22311 (800) 342-2383 (toll-free) www.diabetes.org	Answers questions; provides booklets and materials on diabetes and related care, e.g., medication administration and foot care
American Heart Association	7272 Greenville Avenue Dallas, TX 75231 (800) 242-9721 (toll-free) www.americanheart.org	Provides information and pamphlets on heart problems and related research
American Lung Association	1301 Pennsylvania Avenue NW Suite 800 Washington, DC 20004 (202) 785-3355	Focuses lung health emphasizing clean air and smoke-free living; provides facts about diseases

Name	Address	Type of Assistance
Arthritis Foundation	PO Box 7669 Atlanta, GA 30357 (800) 283-7800 (toll-free) www.arthritis.org	Provides information on and assistance with arthritis
Cancer Information Service	(800) 422-6237 (toll-free)	Provides information about cancer
Family Caregiver Support Group	(NorthWest Senior & Disability Services) (800) 469-8773 (toll-free)	Provides assistance to unpaid family caregivers and grandparents raising grandchildren
Food and Nutrition Information Center	10301 Baltimore Avenue Room 304 Beltsville, MD 20705 (301) 504-5719 www.nal.usda.gov/fnic	Provides credible, accurate, and practical resources for nutrition for health professionals and consumers
National Institute on Aging Information Center	PO Box 8057 Gaithersburg, MD 20898 (800) 222-2225 (toll-free) www.nia.nih.gov	Provides information on popular health topics for older adults
National Mental Health Association	2001 N Beauregard Street 12th Floor Alexandria, VA 22311 (800) 969-6642 (toll-free) www.nmha.org	Provides information and pamphlets on depression and many other areas related to mental health
Quackwatch Inc.	www.quackwatch.org	Makes information available to combat health-related frauds, myths, fads, and fallacies

Networking

PNs will find networking with other nursing professionals to be invaluable. From these professional colleagues you can learn about changes in hospital care as well as community nursing planning. Such a network can be found through membership in professional groups, subscription to organizational publications, or personal interactions at community events and continuing education forums. Find out if your region has a local PN network; such groups often sponsor programs and provide helpful updates about specific programs in the area. If at all possible, attend local and regional meetings, especially when the topics identified for discussion are relevant to your setting.

Reviewing the Toolbox

Looking back into the items available in the PN toolbox, you may be surprised by how well it is stocked. PNs are *accessible* by all communication technology as well as in person. Their *assessments* included formal questionnaires like the congregational health assessment and taking blood pressures with tangible tools. They *planned* with their healthcare committee, the pastoral staff, and ushers for needs that arose. They had *developed* or *intervened* in various ways, such as Jake's establishment of a telephone chain for seniors. Dolores used *evaluation* in formal questions as well as informally when people made comments pertinent to needs and educational programs. Mary's *professional knowledge and background* came through her formal educational programs and her own personal life experiences that enriched her professional judgments. This background helped her become acquainted with *resource* groups and other materials as well as professional networks. Take time to review the tools in your own toolbox. You will be glad for the opportunity to inventory them and identify examples of how you might use them. You probably don't realize how many "tools" you have at your disposal as a PN.

Questions

1. What are some "tools" in your congregation that a PN might use?

2. How is accessibility to people enhanced in your congregation?

3. What are some ways enhanced connections might be developed in your church?

4. How might the tools that a PN in your church uses become more visible and useful?

5. How could some of the PN tools be shared with other churches who don't have a PN?

CHAPTER 6

Providing Educational Health Programs

Parish nurses provide a number of educational programs designed to focus on selected aspects of healthcare. Some relate to maintaining wellness as well as prevention of illness, and others offer general information on healthy lifestyles. Typically an educational program includes a title and objectives (goals to be attained from the program), informational content, some activities for the attendees to do (either physically or mentally), and then a question-and-answer or discussion time related to the content. Finally a written evaluation by the attendees is typically requested to determine if the program addressed the material the attendees wanted to learn.

Programs often are advertised in a way that describes the goals, the importance of the topic, and a brief biography of the presenter reflecting his or her background and expertise. Certainly the advertisement, whether in the form of a printed flyer or online promo via website or social media, needs to include logistics of place and time. Noting that refreshments will be available during the program assures people that the experience is planned to be physically pleasant.

The church community assessment (see Chapter 4) provides a PN with information on what the church members want to learn. With the help of the healthcare team, the PN can then develop a one-year plan for educational programs (see Chapter 4) based on learning priorities identified by parishioners. Such a plan is useful for addressing congregational interests, but it still requires the judgment of the PN and the healthcare team to decide how and when to provide educational experiences on these topics. It is up to the PN to develop each experience in such a way that the presentation is effective. In any teaching or learning situation there are obstacles, such as when students can attend and how long they are able to be involved. PNs need to utilize resource people, and program offerings need to be planned around these challenges. Implementation of the programs is similar to presenting classes in any school experience.

Looking at her one-year plan, Mary determined to focus only on January, and the first workshop identified in the one-year plan was on stress management. Since January was just five weeks away, Mary knew she needed to plan this workshop immediately and contact a resource person. She needed to give careful thought to the presentation. It might be important to have several sessions, one in the morning and another in the evening, with different areas of focus. Then she realized that stress management would necessarily vary according to age and experience levels. At that point, her planning was interrupted by the phone. Three more calls and two drop-in appointments later, Mary had decided that stress was a timely topic for her as well as for others!

Planning for Educational Programs

As you undertake your own planning efforts, consider the stair-step approach outlined on the next page. This approach offers a systematic and intentional way to undertake program design and implementation by beginning with the learners themselves, encompassing the content of learning, considering details related to environment and teaching strategies, and ultimately assessing achievement.

Figure 2 / Stair-Steps in Educational Planning

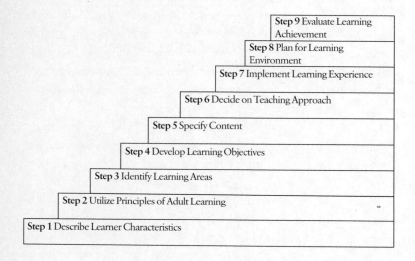

The following Figure 3 expands upon these stair-steps with related terms and examples of each stair-step. Initially it is a challenge to use all these steps in planning for every educational experience, but omitting any one of them may result in disappointing outcomes in the learning experience.

Figure 3 / Expansion of Stair-Steps

Stair-Step	Related Terms	Example
1. Learner Characteristics	Demographic characteristics, educational background, and situational events	Age, sex, culture, years of education; motivation; illness, learning time, and need
2. Principles of Adult Learning	Key concerns in teaching adults	Adults learn best when they are actively involved in pleasant experiences
3. Learning Areas/ Domains	Knowledge Values Performance	Recall; bring together ideas; observe; reflect; recognize; attempt
4. Learning Objectives	Behaviors–Actions Standards Conditions	Identify, make, classify; How many? By when? Using...., with...
5. Content Specification	Identify subject area and what is to be learned	Describe types of depression and treatment
6. Teaching Approaches	Lecture Discussion Demonstration Media Modules	"I am going to present..."; "When would you seek help..."; Show how to do something; Cost, color; Unit of instruction
7. Delivery of Instruction	Art of teaching	Knowledgeable; Organization/clarity; Enthusiasm
8. Learning Environment	Space Chairs Lighting Ventilation Timing	Chairs and tables in room without crowding; Visualization is good; Temperature and air flow; Daytime/evening (short sessions)
9. Evaluation	Questions for small group discussion	Prepare questions related to each objective for the session and have participants respond (they may refer to their notes)

Using the Stair-Steps to Plan

Looking at the nine steps may feel overwhelming. But take a leap of faith and give it a try. Yes, it will require more involvement than merely calling a guest speaker to come to present a session or workshop, but your program will be stronger and more effective if you actually go through the steps. And after the learning experience, the ninth step will offer a basis for determining if the session produced a measurable impact on the participants.

Brief introductory comments for each step are given and followed by Mary's application of the suggestions in her stress management workshop.

Step 1: Describe Learner Characteristics

Learners in a health education program usually will be adults—but that generalization encompasses a wide range in ages, health, and life stage. Contrast the experiences and traits of a twenty-one-year-old with those of an eighty-one-year old! In addition to age itself, key differences might include work history, marital status, parenting stage, education, and health conditions. Learner motivation is also key, and it's a good idea to provide an example at the beginning of your program to help learners personally identify with the content. Another major factor that affects learning is timing. Shorter programs usually maintain better participant attention. The program organizer needs to choose a time in the day or week when participants feel free of other major responsibilities.

Mary realized that she could not accommodate all the differences present in her learner participants, but based on the program times, she might at least bring together participants with somewhat common problems. She could design two sessions—one during the daytime that might be more convenient for retired people and those dealing with illness, and one on a weekday evening or a Saturday for working adults and parents with school-aged children. She could arrange free childcare for the latter session so parents could attend.

Because so many in the congregation had identified the need for an educational program on stress management, Mary decided that motivation would already be high for this topic. She just needed to secure a presenter who was good and could present some useful management techniques.

Step 2: Utilize Principles of Adult Learning

Principles of adult learning include both the art and the science of teaching adults as distinguished from children. For example, rather than giving the adult a lot of information, one principle suggests the teacher needs to help adult learners understand how to use learning resources—particularly how to use the experiences of others as learners engage in discussion with classmates and the teacher (or the presenter, in the case of a workshop). Adult learners do not need an expert to dump a lot of information on them in a single encounter, because retention of new information is limited; more effective is teaching them how to obtain additional information so that, when the need arises, adults will know which resources to access and how to find them.

Another principle of adult learning is to organize the content or activities to be learned within the context of current personal problems. Problem-solving activities enable adults to relate to a given problem and possible solutions to their own personal situations. Another principle is to use participative instructional approaches, with the teacher modeling good behaviors.

An adult learner's self-concept can be affirmed through successful achievement. Breaking content or tasks into small sections so the adult can master each section enhances a sense of personal achievement and competency of knowledge or performance skills. If the teacher is providing content related to relaxation, the examples should be stresses the learner has experienced, and new techniques for relaxation should be presented step by step, allowing time for mastery by the learners and encouragement from the presenter or peers.

Mary tried to apply some of these adult learning principles as she planned workshops on stress. In considering the learning principle on relevancy of the problem, she decided the workshop would be more applicable to the participants if it accommodated some of their personal stress needs. She titled the workshops differently to distinguish the types of stressors to be addressed. "Managing Illness Stressors in Older Adults" was the title for the morning workshop, and "Family Stress Management" was the title for the evening one. Thinking that older adults without young children would attend the morning session and that adults with young families would attend the evening session, Mary reasoned that at least the timing and focus would be relevant for participants from those two groups. Having commonalities in a group would help clarify the workshop focus and direct the experience to participants' needs. She thought about another learning principle—providing participative learning experiences by using problem solving. At first she considered using a panel with persons describing their stresses, but that would only involve panel members. Instead she chose to invite a speaker who would present the information and intersperse the presentation with group discussion related to a specific problem at least twice in an hour.

And one more thing is necessary for adult learners—the workshop should be pleasing. Mary wanted to arrange for healthy beverages and snacks. She consulted with a nutritionist friend to get some inexpensive, healthy snack ideas. (She had only budgeted two hundred dollars for the stress workshop, and that included speaker honoraria.) Maybe if she put together a simple "menu," she could ask some of the workshop participants to bring the food and beverages.

Step 3: Identify Learning Areas
Each learning experience usually includes three kinds of information.

1. New **knowledge** that must be recalled and then pulled together in application

2. **Values** that are observed or reflected by the content
3. **Performance** or skills to practice

Knowledge is often supplied by an expert, whether the PN or a guest speaker. But especially in the congregational context, such knowledge will be received more enthusiastically if connections are made between the spiritual and biblical values of the participants and the health benefits. Just don't forget action steps so that participants leave the event equipped with ideas for implementing their new knowledge and core values.

Mary wanted to include all three learning areas in her program: knowledge that brought together new approaches to use in stress reduction, values that reflected key stressors, and performance that had participants practice using, or at least plan ways they might use, a different approach in coping with their stress. It might be a bit ambitious, but Mary recalled the old maxim, "Nothing ventured, nothing gained."

Step 4: Develop Learning Objectives
The definition of a learning objective is one that specifies the nature and the amount of the desired change in learner behavior. Learning objectives need to include the following attributes:

1. Explicit—use an action verb

2. Measureable—describe observable learner actions

3. Specific—discrete detail; often a number to indicate how many

4. Intentional—striving or attainment; what the learner will achieve

Mary knew, from listening to her teacher friends, that the time to groan was when she developed objectives, because most people did. But she decided that putting a few words on paper did not have to be so hard.

1. Identify what stress is, in thirty words or less.

2. Describe six events that produce stress.

3. Make a list of six things to do to manage stress.

4. Illustrate the use of stress reduction approaches by using one of the workshop suggestions for managing stress in an anecdotal situation.

a. Family conflict over Saturday activities (Family Group)

b. Older adult managing high glucose level (Older Adult with Illness Group)

The exercise only took Mary ten minutes, and upon reviewing her work, she noted that she had action words, observable actions, specific numbers, and conditions to be achieved in the workshop. Mary gave herself a well-deserved pat on the back.

Step 5: Specify Content

There is so much to learn that it is often no simple task to divide a learning experience into parts that all learners will deal with easily. If there is too much information, most learners feel overwhelmed, but if there is too little information, the quick learner will become disinterested. It may help to map content out, and you may find that, by conceiving real-life situations with desired results, the objectives outlined in Step 4 help to distill the breadth of potential information into well-defined content.

That was the case for Mary, who decided that for the stress workshop the content might be mapped out as follows:

1. Definition of stress

2. Examples of stressful experiences

3. Approaches to reduce stress

4. Practice using techniques to minimize hurtful stress

Out of the wide world of what to include about stress—from the old "fight or flight" description to the myriad potential human stressors—her objectives clarified the type and number of approaches to use, and actually helped specify her content. In fact, Mary had the brainstorm of using a summary of those objectives in her promotion of the workshop. By offering people a concise, action-oriented description of the experience, they would know what to expect—and should be able to evaluate the effectiveness of the workshop based on its ability to deliver on that description.

Step 6: Decide on Teaching Approach

Traditionally the teacher or presenter lectured, and the learners listened and took notes. But a lot of adult learners no longer like to take notes, even on their laptops or tablets. While some presenters try to address that trend by providing handouts or using PowerPoint presentations and other audiovisual aids, the average adult learner will prefer an interactive experience. Be sure to allow time and space for discussion of open-ended questions, and to invite questions from the participants themselves. Such verbal interaction with the content can easily lead to problem-solving activities. (Another creative teaching approach is the module, which is presented later in this chapter.)

When Mary reached this step in her planning, she reviewed available approaches. She quickly settled on an expert presentation, combined with a discussion. She did not have enough budget to get a quality DVD on the subject, so she decided that an effective speaker would demonstrate how to use the stress management approaches. She would consult with her healthcare committee members and ask them for recommendations. A good psychologist could present the background information, and then participants could divide into small groups to discuss in depth some of their stressful experiences.

Step 7: Implement Learning Experience

An old educational research study compared teacher ratings for two different teachers. Teacher A was always rated highly by the students, even though he primarily cracked jokes and entertained the students; in contrast, Teacher B, who presented excellent content but had a less animated style of presentation, was rated poorly. The lesson? Enthusiasm is key for every teacher. Of course, an entertaining presentation needs to be coupled with accurate facts and well-organized knowledge.

With these factors in mind, Mary knew she wanted to find a presenter who did more than research; she wanted the expert to have hands-on experience with implementing practical strategies for stress management. And if he or she had a decent sense of humor and a genuine passion for engaging with people, that was all the better! She wanted someone who could be enthusiastic about reducing stress—not a person who spoke in a monotone and presented information without interacting with the participants.

Step 8: Plan for Learning Environment
Five points need to be considered with respect to the place where learning is to occur:

1. Space—Elbow room for people
2. Chairs—Reasonably comfortable seating for all who attend
3. Lighting—Adequate general lighting in all areas of the room; some outside light is preferred
4. Ventilation—Heating and cooling must be considered, along with airflow, to keep learners alert
5. Timing—Not only the time of day but also the duration of the presentation; do not plan more than thirty minutes of presentation without a change of pace, including questions or discussion

In order to plan appropriately in each of these areas, Mary realized that she should probably have some process for preregistration or sign-up. That way, she could reserve space and request room accommodations suited to the registered participants. While she was it, she decided to include a question on the registration form about whether childcare was needed, especially for the family workshop. She also made a mental note to ensure that the workshop space for the older adults would be accessible for her seniors and in reasonable proximity to the restrooms.

Step 9: Evaluate Learning Achievement

Real evaluation involves more than the quick "Good workshop!" comment from participants. True learning achievement is most clearly assessed by questions. Because questions are often considered "windows to the mind," it is important to have several questions related to each objective of any given presentation. Learners in a workshop-style experience probably prefer to respond to questions in a discussion rather than a written format. Even though only one person can respond at a time, each response provides the presenter and other workshop participants feedback as to how a particular responder processed the presented information. Some participants might have responded differently, and based on the way the presenter interacts with another participant's response, they can learn if they had processed the information accurately.

Mary realized that if all participants could accomplish at least one of the stated objectives—to describe six new approaches to use in managing personal stress—then she would know it had been a successful workshop. It would be appropriate to ask participants to share those approaches in the group at the conclusion of the event. Of course, whether they actually implemented the approaches would be up to them!

Because she wanted to collect as much feedback on the overall experience as possible, however, Mary decided to also prepare a brief written evaluation form. She chose a distinctive colored paper so it would be easy to distinguish and retrieve any that might be left on the tables. On the evaluation form each objective should be listed and then the person completing the evaluation can comment on how well she or he was able to achieve the objective. A few questions should be included about the speaker's presentation approach and inclusion of sufficient content. Logistical questions about workshop timing, the classroom, and the refreshments provide information regarding how "pleasant" the workshop was for the participants. It may be helpful to have participants identify suggestions for other workshops on related topics. (The evaluation form Mary prepared for the stress workshop is included as Appendix F.)

Workshop Logistics

Of course, after completing the stair-steps of the educational staircase, there will still be administrative details to consider and practical follow-up steps to take. Consider a few from the list that follows. Depending on the nature of your program, you may have fewer details—or more of them!

■ If not already done, develop a budget and secure approval from appropriate committees or leaders.

■ Solicit recommendations for expert presenters.

■ Contact potential presenter and ascertain required honorarium or other expenses (e.g., mileage, meals).

■ Finalize menu and arrange for purchase and preparation of food and beverages.

■ Reserve space and request any special configuration of the room (e.g., number and arrangement of chairs).

■ Confirm access to technology as needed (e.g., sound system, projector for showing PowerPoint slides).

■ Recruit needed volunteers (for promotion, registration, setup, cleanup, "hosting," etc.).

■ Promote the event both in the congregation (bulletin, website, newsletter, bulletin board) and in the community (flyers, newspaper, radio).

■ Prepare handouts for workshop participants as appropriate. (See "Workshop Program Handout" at http://www.judsonpress.com/ free_download_book_excerpts.cfm.)

■ Prepare a sign-in sheet (which can ask for contact information from all participants); also have nametags available.

Building an Educational Module

Not every health-related issue will lend itself to a presentation-discussion format, with a single presenter addressing a focused topic. Some issues are multifaceted and require a more complex and nuanced approach. For those topics, a module approach to congregational and community education might be ideal.

A module is defined as a unit of instruction. Thus, a module approach to teaching would approach one issue from multiple perspectives—or multiple related issues in different segments or units. This approach can be a useful strategy for exploring controversial issues because it allows a topic to be considered from a biblical-ethical perspective in one workshop, from a physiological perspective in another, and from a relational-emotional perspective in a third. It might also be used to mine multiple strategies for a significant health concern. For example, a module approach to heart health might feature units on nutrition, exercise, medication, and stress management.

When Jake got a call from Pastor Susan about church members who were asking him questions about alternative medicine and a holistic healing, Jake knew that a traditional workshop with a single presenter would barely scratch the surface of such an issue. No single resource or expert could cover it all, particularly when opinions about non-Western medicine and therapies varied so widely even (and especially) within the healthcare community. A module approach seemed to be the only one to take.

Jake started by doing some preliminary research on his own, consulting the Internet and medical libraries as well as professional nursing journals and other publications. Then he asked his regional PN network about local experts in the area who might be able to address the questions and concerns, not only from a medical perspective but also from a religious and theological one. After all, many alternative therapies and forms of Eastern medicine had roots in or connections to non-Christian belief systems.

Then Jake connected with some church members recommended by Pastor Sue. These members had some experience in homeopathic remedies, both as complementary treatments to traditional Western medicine and as alternative treatments. The conversations Jake had with those folks were particularly helpful in crafting an outline of the key questions and issues a typical church member might have about the efficacy, risks, and orthodoxy of such treatments—without getting entangled in the complexities of research and data.

In developing a module approach to teaching, the PN will go through a planning process similar to the stair-step approach. See the Building Modules section.

Building Modules

1. Purpose Statement—Indicates reason for development

2. Preview—Specifies background data and module content so that the learner can determine whether he or she needs to study prior to attending the module session

3. Objectives—Describe action and performance behaviors; what the learner does

4. Equipment and Materials—Identify items needed while studying module

5. Design of Instruction—Indicates how the learner is to proceed through materials

6. Presentation of Instructional Content—Learning sequence which usually is self-contained

7. Learning Activities—Indicate learner interaction with content

8. Self-Tests—Indicate whether the learner is learning material included in a given objective (these typically are short questions interspersed throughout the written material)

9. References—List of supplemental materials included in a file that expand the learner's perspective

Jake carved out a block of uninterrupted time and space to plan his first module program. He determined to focus his process on selected complementary and alternative medicine (CAM) therapies. His goal was to have written materials available to give to people whenever they came to Pastor Sue or to him with questions about whether to begin some non-Western medical treatment.

By the end of the day Jake was amazed with what he had written. As soon as he edited it, he made a copy for Pastor Sue, inviting her input and revisions. (See "Module—Introduction to CAM Therapies" at http://www.judsonpress.com/free_download_book_excerpts.cfm.)

The simple approach to providing an educational program is to call a speaker to present a given topic and invite participants. However, such a loose approach may not justify the speaker honorarium or the participants' time if minimal learning occurs. Using the Stair-Step approach, ensures a way to plan effective adult learning experiences in such a way that learning achievement is measureable. The use of these steps is illustrated in the development of an educational workshop and a learning module, two of the most common educational approaches the PN may use.

Questions
1. How might an educational program plan be used at your church, with or without a PN to implement it?

2. Which of the points of the educational plan seem most essential? Why?

3. If a health-related workshop is needed in your church, how would an educational plan help in designing it?

4. Can you think of any health areas for which an educational module would benefit your church community?

5. How might some educational background help a PN in providing health education?

6. What might a teacher, teamed up with a nurse, contribute to developing some educational programs?

CHAPTER 7

Age-Related Health Needs, Considering Religious Values and Beliefs

PNs need to consider common health problems that occur at different stages of life in order to comprehensively plan for these needs as they arise. Both preventive and health-promoting activities need to be included with respect to potential illnesses. (Typical illnesses are almost general knowledge; for example, children have communicable diseases, adults have neurological problems such as Parkinson's, and older people have strokes and heart attacks. Lists can be found in most family or life cycle websites and articles.)

The PN needs to focus on religious values and beliefs that may accompany age-related illnesses and needs. Trying to integrate these values and beliefs with the presence of illness or health needs often generates many questions that need to be discussed.

Consider the following outline of common health-related issues, grouped by age range. The parish nurse may be called upon to educate or advise parishioners on any and all of these matters, and more.

I. Infants and Children (0–12)

    A. Circumcision

    B. Immunizations

    C. Developmental delays and milestones

    D. Age of accountability

    E. Gender identity

    F. Social skills

    G. Childhood obesity

    H. Special needs

        1. Physical disabilities

        2. Emotional and mental disabilities, including autism spectrum

        3. Learning disabilities

II. Teens (13–19)

    A. Work and service

    B. Peer relationships

        1. Friendships and dating

        2. Virtual interactions (social media, texting, online gaming, cyber bullying)

        3. Sexual identity and expression

        4. Pregnancy and sexually transmitted diseases (STDs, including HIV/AIDS)

    C. Puberty and adolescence (physical, emotional, and social development)

    D. Depression and suicide risk

    E. Addictions

III. Young Adults (18–35)

    A. Relationships

        1. Singleness

        2. Friendships and dating

        3. Attaining independence (financial and emotional)

4. Changing relationships with family
B. Education and Employment
    1. Discerning God's will and direction
    2. Student debt
    3. Unemployment and underemployment

IV. Adults (21–65)
A. Career
    1. Livable wage versus meaningful work
    2. Vocational opportunities and transitions
    3. Balancing work, family, and faith
B. Relationships and sexuality
    1. Dating and marriage
    2. Divorce
    3. Remarriage
    4. Changing hormone levels and sexual function
C. Pregnancy and infertility
    1. Contraception and family planning
    2. Infertility and treatments
    3. Adoption
D. Parenting
    1. First-time parents
    2. Parenting a child with special needs
    3. Parenting in blended or stepfamilies
    4. Young adult children, including "boomerang" children
    5. Adult children of aging parents

V. Seniors (65+)
A. Physical health (Because of the number of chronic illnesses occurring in older adults, a few of the most common areas of concern are listed.)
    1. Heart conditions
    2. Strokes and after effects (partial paralysis)

3. Diabetes

4. Hypertension

5. Arthritis and other mobility issues

6. Cancer

7. Osteoporosis

B. Emotional and mental health

  1. Dementia

  2. Loneliness

  3. Depression

  4. Anger (over chronic health issues and life challenges)

  5. Grief and fear of death

  6. End-of-life decisions (including advanced directives)

Dolores sighed when she finished reviewing the list of health concerns likely to confront her in congregational ministry. She could imagine the questions that might arise as church members tried to apply their Christian faith to these complex and personal issues. She would be sure to encourage people to find a good family doctor and stay current with annual physicals and self-exams. Then she could focus on the spiritual and faith-based aspects of the health-related concerns. Even then, the list of concerns was overwhelming. Where to begin?

Dolores decided to consult her pastor about which health issues he thought were of primary concern for the congregation. Rev. Carter responded in writing with an encouraging e-mail, applauding Dolores for the time and insight she had already invested in the discernment process. The pastor suggested several key areas for focus, if not in the first year, then in the first five years of the parish nurse's ministry.

■ Talk with Sister Jackie about health aspects that interface with religious beliefs and practices of teens.

■ See if you can identify a speaker for a workshop for young parents.

■ Contact several of our seniors to ask for "insider" input on identifying their priority needs.

Dolores was grateful to Rev. Carter for his prompt and encouraging response. She was surprised that compared to hers, his list didn't really look too bad! Clearly, God meant to affirm her efforts through the pastor's helpful words. Energized anew, she got right to work on his suggestions.

Teen Issues

Today's teenagers face many issues that offer significant opportunities to put faith in conversation through concrete questions of physical, emotional, and mental health. Adolescence is a time when bodies and minds are developing rapidly as children make the transition into adulthood—and their physical development usually outpaces their psycho-emotional maturity. The PN will want to work closely not only with the pastor or youth director, but also in communication with parents in approaching educational programs for teens. Find out what the church leadership and parents have identified as key biblical teachings and faithful practice, especially as they relate to such matters as dating, sexual identity, and sexual behavior. Be respectful of those convictions, even as you may offer a different perspective based on medical research and professional experience. What education has already occurred, and what areas do the parents or youth director feel ill-equipped to tackle?

When Dolores met with Sister Jackie, the youth director at her church, Jackie explained that in talking to the teens about sexual issues she had used 1 Corinthians 6:19, the Scripture that focuses on our body being God's temple, and Romans 12:1, which talks about being transformed and renewing our minds. Of course, the teens still had many concerns about their emerging sexual desires and the spiritual and physical effects of their decisions, including STDs. Jackie invited Dolores to come to one of the youth group meetings to meet the teens and field some of their questions.

When Dolores met with the teens, she found that they were really thinking about their sexuality—about who they were as sexual beings and how their choices affected their relationships with God and other people. Dolores could answer some of the questions they asked, but she told them she would have to get back to them on some others! After the meeting Dolores and Sister Jackie talked about how to deal with some of the issues being raised. They decided to consult with parents of young adults, whose children were no longer in the youth group. Some of those parents might be able to act as mentors to the teens themselves or to the teens' parents, offering them the wisdom of experience in how to deal with these issues.

Parenting Years

While Dolores's pastor had suggested a workshop for "young parents," what PNs like Dolores may soon discover is that, among adults ranging as widely in age from late teens to early fifties, a common concern is coping with parenting while *also* trying to care for their own aging parents. These are often busy years in a given family unit, with school and extracurricular activities, working parents, and church and community commitments, and then suddenly the same parent needs to take over the caregiving of his or her own aging parents.

That was what Dolores discovered when she went to a parishioner's house to assist a distraught mother with lice treatment for her eight-year-old daughter. Dolores knew it wasn't really her role to handle the hair washing and house cleaning that were necessary, but she could stop by to offer a compassionate ear and professional advice. Over a glass of iced tea, Dolores learned that it wasn't just the horror and guilt of a lice infestation that was overwhelming Helen, the thirty-something-year-old mother of two. It was also the care of a father-in-law in the early stages of dementia.

Dolores took the time first to assure Helen that head lice weren't the result of poor parenting; then she put Helen in touch with another church member who had recently dealt with a lice infestation of her own. The other mother was immediately sympathetic and offered to come later that day to help with the laundry and housecleaning.

That left Dolores with the task of offering to research resources that might support Helen (and other parishioners like her) in juggling the demands of raising school-aged children with the need to care for increasingly dependent aging parents. More than a workshop on Christian parenting, Dolores relayed to Rev. Carter at the next staff meeting that she thought a seminar about honoring one's aging parents through care and wise counsel might be a higher priority. Rev. Carter agreed.

Older Adult Needs

Older adults typically develop problems with mobility, confusion, or chronic illness. It is best for them if they can manage these changes in their own homes. Some older adults have a lot of personal resources and creativity, while others rely on others to help them. Most learn new coping techniques, adjust to their problems happily, and live very productive and useful lives. Parish nurses need to be attentive to concerns they hear about older adults, and then help to develop programs to meet those expressed needs.

As people age, they begin to experience social isolation. Their own children grow up and move out—often away from the town where they were raised. Spouses and friends begin to die. Other friends move to distant locations, whether into assisted living communities or smaller and less expensive homes, or to be closer to family members. Even in reasonably healthy and active seniors, physical changes often mean less ability to drive at night or keep up with the volunteer work or travel they once enjoyed. Recognition of those limitations, combined with an awareness of their own mortality, often means that the increasingly isolated elder parishioners feel alone and downcast at the changes age has brought.

When Dolores began to ask some of her older parishioners about their biggest health-related concerns, the issue of loneliness—and in too many instances, depression—was indeed at the top of the list. But it was not the only issue. Other seniors mentioned a desire for *less* activity, especially those who were helping to care for grandchildren or who were supporting a spouse, an adult child, or other family member with some type of health challenge or life crisis.

When Dolores shared her observations with her PN colleague, Nina nodded. "I've found the same dynamics among the seniors at our church. I've started to use an illustration that one of our more active and insightful older members designed. It's based on Psalm 1, especially verse 3, which says about the righteous, 'They are like trees planted by streams of water, which yield their fruit in its season, and their leaves do not wither. In all that they do, they prosper.' It's a picture of a tree, with one side withered with bare branches labeled with words such as *loneliness, grief,* and *helplessness.* The other side of the tree has healthy leaves and positive words like *meaning, hope,* and *wisdom* penciled among the leaves. It's a powerful picture of the two sides of growing older—or what the artist likes to call 'gaining maturity.'"

"Would you send me a copy of it?" Dolores asked. "It sounds like it could be a helpful way to keep the complex issues of aging in perspective. How have you used it in your ministry?"

Nina described a Bible study for older adults that the artist had led on the topic of maturity, both physical and spiritual. "I've also used it in my own planning for educational programs on older adult concerns. It has been a great visual to make sure that our programs are balanced with positive experiences as well as addressing issues of real concern." Dolores thought a study by and for her senior parishioners might be a great way to not only foster spiritual maturity, but to also address the sense of social isolation so many older adults experience. It would also offer more positive content for learners, taking their focus off of aging bodies and decreasing independence.

Figure 4 on page 87 depicts the tree illustration described by Mary. How might its labels suggest other programs or events to nurture, encourage, and connect older adults in your congregation? Education need not be focused exclusively on physical or mental health. Many older adults would appreciate church-sponsored trips that would connect them to history and culture, or small groups offering a chance to teach and learn new hobbies or skills. And by engaging in those experiences, participants will also be meeting real social, emotional, and psychological needs. Consider programs sponsored by other organizations as well, such as Shepherd Center Central's "Adventures in Learning" programs (see http://sccentral.org). Such organizations often hold their events in churches or other houses of worship, and the programs are open to the community.

Of course, older adults also have pressing health challenges that a PN can address in helpful ways. A workshop on advanced directives, long-term care insurance, and estate planning would be educational—and might offer an opportunity to address the intergenerational concerns of younger adult members stressed about ensuring care for their aging parents. Programs related to specific chronic illnesses and common prescription medications might require the support of other medical experts, such as a church member who is a retired physician or the parishioner who works as researcher for a pharmaceutical company.

Health needs occur throughout the life cycle. The PN is able to help integrate the physical and emotional aspects of these needs with religious values. Some of these issues present questions about the choices people need to make regarding suggested steps in treatment or plans for care. For example, is there a biblical or theological requirement for Christian parents to have their son circumcised? Does an adult child violate the commandment to honor his or her father and mother by sending an aging parent to a care facility rather than personally providing care? A major goal of the PN is to plan educational experiences and, as needed, to provide individual counseling, sometimes in conjunction with clergy, to help parishioners with translating biblical principles to life-cycle needs and healthcare decisions.

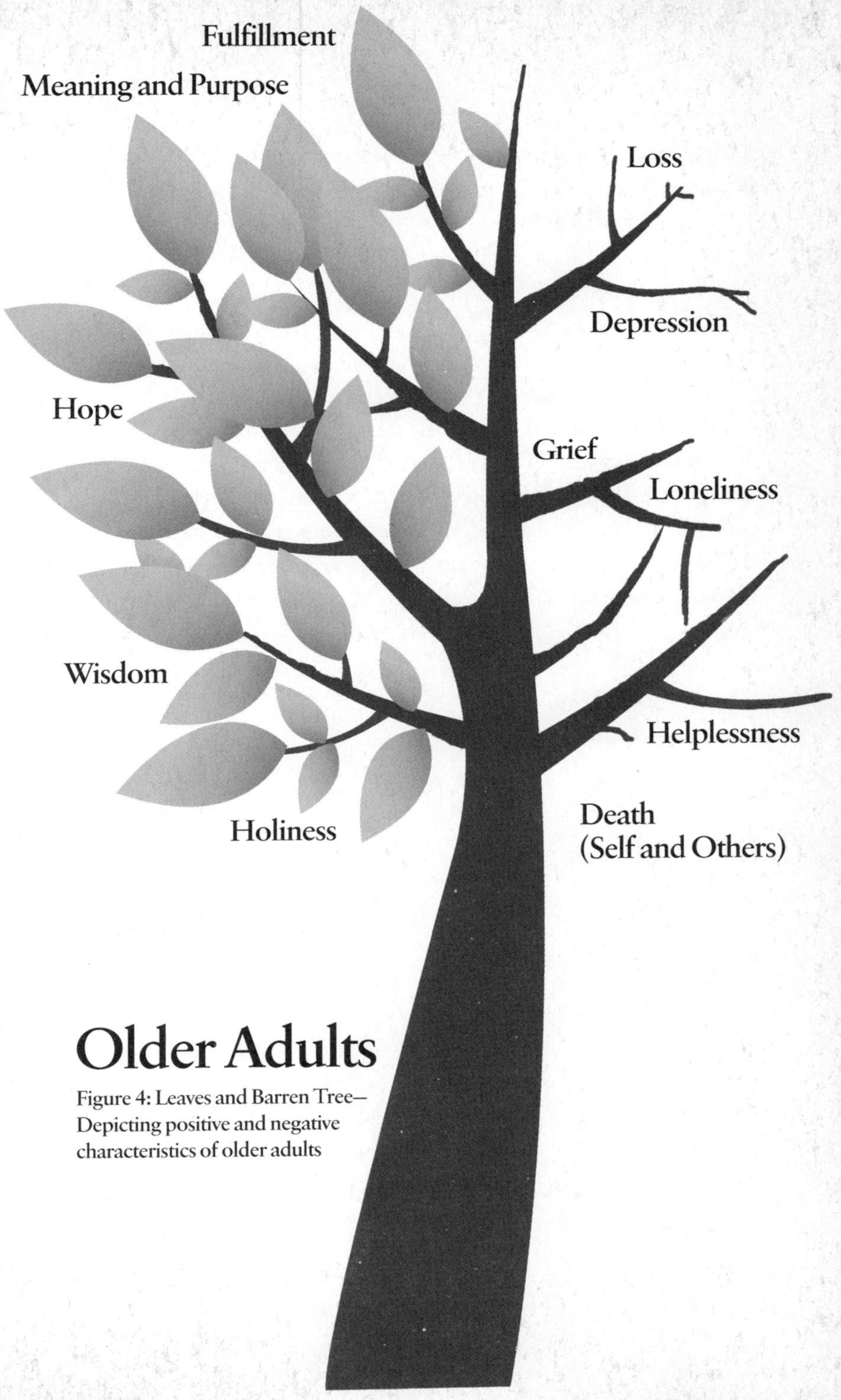

Fulfillment

Meaning and Purpose

Loss

Depression

Hope

Grief

Loneliness

Wisdom

Helplessness

Holiness

Death
(Self and Others)

Older Adults

Figure 4: Leaves and Barren Tree—
Depicting positive and negative
characteristics of older adults

Questions

1. List two questions you have that relate to religious values and the following age groups:

A. Infants and Children

B. Teens

C. Young Adults

D. Adults

E. Seniors

2. When have members of your congregation asked you about a religious value(s) related to a health issue they might be dealing with?

3. Think of three different periods in your life, and give an example of a faith-based health issue you experienced at each period.

4. What are the priority issues you would identify for your congregation, as Dolores and Rev. Carter identified for theirs? Why?

5. What other topics would you add to the content outlined in this chapter?

CHAPTER 8

Caring for Individual Health Needs in Varied Locaions

While traditionally people go to healthcare facilities, such as clinics or hospitals, to seek medical care, in the Gospels we see Jesus modeling a healing ministry whenever he encountered people in need. Some, like the woman with a bleeding issue and the man whose son was ill, came to him. As he traveled from place to place, visiting private homes, Jesus also healed acquaintances, friends, and family members, such as Peter's mother-in-law. And in the parable of the Good Samaritan, Jesus illustrated a model for healing ministry "along the way"—attending to an immediate need on the roadside and then arranging for longer-term care with the promise of follow-up. So also, the parish nurse will come across people in varied locations with diverse needs who require different types of care—physical, emotional, spiritual, and mental.

In the Church Office

Clergy, ministerial leadership, administrative office staff, custodians, and others spend a lot of time at church, as paid employees and as volunteers. These individuals each have their own physical, mental, and emotional health concerns, which may be heightened during stressful times in the life of the church. As in any other profession, tension between staff members, crises in the organizational finances, and conflicts among leaders and members about ministry vision and priorities are all a part of church life. Such stressors take a toll, physically and emotionally. And because many church staffs become something like a family, staff members sense one another's concerns and needs.

A PN brings professional expertise to fellow church staff members and their health needs too. That may involve casual conversations that touch on questions about preventing the spread of viruses around the office, or debates about the latest trend in diet or exercise. It may also include discreet requests to meet privately with the PN to discuss matters of a more personal nature—a troubling diagnosis, a bothersome symptom, or a challenging situation with a family member, parishioner, or colleague. Such interactions are opportunities for the PN to support the larger ministry team even as the team members, in their own areas of ministry and gifting, support the work of the PN.

One day during her office hours, Mary encountered the youth pastor, Tom, who had come to work with a headache that rapidly escalated to a fever. After urging him to go to the doctor immediately, Mary later heard that Tom was admitted to the hospital and diagnosed with a serious infection. Thank God she had been around to advise immediate intervention! Mary was also able to coordinate with Tom's adult volunteers to ensure that well-meaning youth didn't drop by to visit—disturbing Tom's rest and risking contagion themselves.

Nina was walking past the restroom after a meeting one afternoon when she heard a commotion inside. It was divine providence that she arrived in time to assist with emergency first aid for the aging church secretary, who had become light-headed and taken a fall. Nina stayed with Señora Claudia until the EMTs arrived, and then Nina called Claudia's nephew to meet her at the emergency room. "Your *tia* should be fine," Nina assured him, "but you'll want to be there to talk with the doctors and to make sure she gets home safely."

Before and After Church Services

Of course, it isn't only in the church office during regularly scheduled office hours that the PN will meet people who have health concerns. In fact the church building itself, before or after worship services, is one of the most common places to interact with the PN. The coffee pot during fellowship hour is akin to the water cooler in a corporate environment. People may be simply socializing, sharing the joys and sorrows of the week, retelling highlights of some Christian service opportunity or reviewing the Sunday school discussion or the sermon. But upon seeing the PN enter, a parishioner's thoughts might immediately turn to health, especially if he or she has a particular question or concern. Some church members who feel reluctant to call for an appointment with the PN will find that the informality of the coffee hour provides an easy opportunity to ask a question or describe a concern.

In such cases, the PN will need to use discretion to decide whether the particular health concern can be appropriately addressed in such an informal and public context. Sometimes even recounting the problem causes the parishioner to become emotional, drawing the attention and concern of others. Carrying on a prolonged discussion in the social room is difficult, even in a quiet corner; when privacy is needed, the PN may need to ask the parishioner to schedule an office visit to explore the concern properly. Other times, the concern is more immediate, but the PN will want to identify accommodations that ensure safety and space for someone who may be experiencing light-headedness, pain, or a panic attack. Such accommodations may require a chair, a couch, some cool water, or breathing room.

Dolores arrived early for the Sunday service and headed for the fellowship hall for coffee. She had barely filled her cup when Sharon approached with a stricken look on her face. "The doctor says I need to have a hysterectomy. But we would like to have more children, and—I have so many questions!" She stopped abruptly as her eyes filled with tears.

Dolores reached out to Sharon and squeezed her hand. "Oh, this is a hard one. Let's go somewhere we can talk more privately for a few minutes."

When they reached an empty classroom, Dolores listened as Sharon poured out her confusion, grief, and fear. It wasn't only the desire for more children that upset her; she was fearful about a diagnosis dire enough to make such surgery necessary. And she was worried about how such a major procedure would alter her body and her identity as a woman. Dolores took the time to talk with her, touching on each concern—physical, emotional, and spiritual—assuring her that God wouldn't object to a life-saving surgery, no matter how major, and that a woman was still very much a woman with or without a uterus. Then she offered to meet with Sharon in the next few days so that Dolores could address any medical issues related to the diagnosis and recommended surgery.

Sharon agreed. "I'm just so glad I bumped into you this morning. I've been so worried and upset that I didn't even want to come to church today. Thanks for listening. I feel a little more like worshipping now that I know you're available to help me walk through these decisions!" The two women hugged and then hurried to join the rest of the congregation in the sanctuary.

Jake was gathering his coat and Bible when Trent rushed over to him. "Have you got a minute? I wanted to ask you about why my blood sugar may be running higher."

"Sure, I have time. What's going on with your diabetes?" Jake gestured to the pew and the two men sat down together. The sanctuary was emptying quickly, so they had a measure of privacy in which to talk.

"For this past week my levels have been up about thirty points every evening, and I don't know why. I'm exercising about the same, and I'm not under any particular stress."

Jake nodded. He and Trent had previously identified stress and heavy exercise as risk factors for heightened blood sugar. "What about your diet? Are you eating more fruit than usual? I know I have been. Peaches and cherries are in season right now!" Jake grinned.

"You're right! I've been enjoying a lot more fresh fruit lately. I hadn't thought about that affecting my levels because fruit is so healthy."

"Unfortunately, even natural sugars will have an impact on someone with diabetes mellitus," Jake frowned sympathetically. "You don't have to give up the fruit; just reduce your carbohydrates if you want to increase your fruit. But if you do so and you don't see an immediate drop in your levels, you should definitely see your doctor."

Note that Jake was able to address Trent's concerns with a few minutes of conversation, while Dolores needed additional privacy to attend to Sharon and offered to follow up with an office appointment if Susan desired. Both PNs, however, were willing to take the time right then and there to respond to the questions and concerns of the parishioners.

Home

For most people, home is the place most favored for releasing their inhibitions and being themselves. What better place for ministry to happen? Ideally, the parish nurse is able to take his or her ministry to the church members by visiting them in the comfort and familiarity of their own homes.

Home settings provide helpful windows into the experiences of those in the home. When illness strikes a household, the home's usual relaxed atmosphere often changes because the illness affects both the sick person and the caregivers. If you have ever been caregiver to a seriously ill person, you will understand this dynamic on a different level, but the PN will also become sensitive to the changes. These changes happen in concrete, tangible ways, such as lighting levels, volume of conversation and activity, scents and odors, and cleanliness. Changes also occur in the atmosphere of the home—in the relational dynamics, the rhythm of life, and the emotional and psychological vitality of all family members. Such changes may become symptoms in and of themselves, helping an attentive PN evaluate the overall health of the household.

When Mary visited the Conner home, it was in response to a call from a wife desperately concerned about her husband. "He isn't eating," Caryn confided as Mary entered the home. "I'm afraid that he's given up on life." On entering the bedroom where George was watching TV from his wheelchair, Mary understood the other woman's concern. The room was dim, the TV volume was barely audible, and George seemed to be staring into space.

Intentionally, Mary went straight to the curtains and pulled them aside to let sunlight flood the room. While she did so, she greeted George brightly and didn't pull any punches. "Hi! I hear you've lost your appetite. What's going on? I know it isn't Caryn's cooking!"

George shrugged. "I think the meds take my appetite away." He was undergoing treatment for an inoperable brain tumor.

Caryn offered to set up tray tables in the bedroom for everyone and started for the door. Mary stopped her. "Let's eat in the kitchen. I'll help George get to the table while you get the food, OK?" The PN wanted to get him out of the bedroom and into a different space. She knew that too much sameness in routine and environment had a tendency to feed depression.

Over lunch, they talked about the flowers in the backyard and the birds at the birdbath. And before she left, Mary encouraged both Caryn and George to continue having him at the table for meals. "It will be a good change of scenery for you, George, and easier on Caryn if she doesn't have to prepare the meal and carry everything back and forth to the bedroom."

From just an hour or so in the home, Mary had observed that it wasn't only George who was suffering; as his caregiver, Caryn also needed encouragement and little moments of respite from her responsibilities. Sharing a meal at the table restored some normalcy to the relationship for both of them. And hopefully, it would help both spouses to consider other little things they could do to make life better, easier, and brighter for the other person.

As she drove home, Mary made a mental note to call her PN friend Dolores. If she remembered correctly, Dolores had helped her church start a support group for long-term caregivers, including a respite program so individual caregivers could get away for an hour or so at a time. She thought Caryn would really benefit from involvement in that kind of group.

Dolores was delighted at the prospect of welcoming someone from a neighboring church to their group. "And don't you also have a list of volunteers willing to run errands for homebound church members? You might want to put Caryn in touch with someone on that list. The volunteer might be willing to stay with the husband while Caryn runs the errands—or at least to linger for a brief visit when dropping off the errand items."

Hospital and Rehabilitation

A very tangible activity for the PN is visiting people in the hospital and at rehabilitation centers. Whenever possible, a home visit prior to scheduled surgery will provide a PN with background information about how the family is preparing for the surgical experience and if they have any special fears or needs. Don't hesitate to pray with the family regarding their particular concerns. And as appropriate or desired, alert the pastor or other church leaders about the parishioner's medical procedure so that the minister can make a pastoral visit, either prior to surgery, before discharge, or during convalescence and recovery.

At the hospital the PN can consult with the medical team to get the general plan for care, expected prognosis, and any special equipment—such as walkers, shower benches, or commodes (bedside toilets)—that might be needed during recovery. Visiting in the hospital also allows the PN to assess the patient's baseline of physical mobility, emotional response, and spiritual concerns.

Equipped with such information, the PN can discern what kind of additional support the family might need, such as help with meals, childcare, errands, or caregiver support. The PN can also help the family determine what home preparations might be needed, such as moving beds and chairs, removing scatter rugs, or obtaining special foods.

Some parishioners will be quick to involve their PN in the process of planning for or following up on hospitalizations and rehabilitation. Nina was thrilled when Señora Nuñez called her on Monday to tell her about Señor Nuñez's cardiac surgery to install a pacemaker, which was scheduled for Thursday. Señora Nuñez had boasted of the PN to the cardiology nurse, who had asked to speak with Nina about some of the post-surgical needs the family might have. Nina accompanied Señor and Señora Nuñez to their pre-surgical appointment on Wednesday and took careful notes on the cardiology nurse's instructions. On Thursday morning, Nina stopped by the hospital surgical waiting room to encourage Señora Nuñez during the long wait. She reminded the older woman to call her with the surgeon's report and with details about when Señor Nuñez would be discharged. Nina wanted to be there to assist with settling Señor Nuñez back into the home—after confirming that Señora Nuñez had made all the necessary accommodations for his convalescence.

Following the model Jesus provided of encountering sick people in many places, the PN can offer guidance in health promotion and prevention of additional illness in multiple settings—office, hospital or home. As the examples in this chapter illustrate, the PN often meets parishioners in the hospital to encourage them during long periods of waiting or in preparation for transition to home. In the home setting the nursing observations of the condition of the sick person as well as home environmental adaptations are often needed and welcomed. The church office or other locations prior to or following a service help parishioners and/or family unburden their minds about health concerns so they are free to worship God.

Questions

1. Where might church members be most likely to encounter a PN in your church? Why?

2. What experiences have you had with nursing outside of a doctor's office or hospital (e.g., community or school nurse, visiting nurse, home care or hospice nursing)?

3. What questions might a caregiver want to ask a PN visiting the caregiver's home?

4. What might a PN learn from a visit to your home? What added perspective can the family members gain from the PN's observations or advice?

5. Have you ever known someone who had to be hospitalized again within a day or two after initially being discharged? What might a post-surgical home visit from a PN have accomplished to prevent such a return?

6. If someone in your home has had surgery, what questions did you or your family have about the care details or the surgery that you would have liked to talk about with a PN?

CHAPTER 9

Health Promotion Programs for Special Needs

The Hebrew term *shalom* connotes a sense of wholeness that provides the conceptual basis for health promotion. In the second chapter of 3 John, the writer prays that we would prosper in health. Wholeness and health need to be of particular focus in the church. One organization that models a health focus is the Centers for Disease Control and Prevention (CDC), which targets key problem areas based on statistical and other data. The CDC updates a list of areas every ten years under the title "Healthy People." Thirteen new topic areas were added for the most recent list, "Healthy People 2020."

The Healthy People 2020 list consists of major health problems occurring in the United States. Measureable goals are developed to promote health in each area so that the nation's progress can be tracked. For example, the area of nutrition is included in both the 2010 and 2020 lists (with "overweight" changed to "weight status" for 2020). Population statistics are compiled according to specific parameters for measuring weight status and obesity. During the ten-year period, programs and activities are initiated to promote healthy nutrition and to reduce the number of people who are overweight. For instance, one current program is directed toward modifying school lunches to include more fruits and vegetables. Another step to improve nutrition for children is to remove the soft drinks and candy bars from school vending machines. It is hoped that when statistics are next obtained, the previously frightening increase in overweight children will show some evidence of decrease.

Much of medicine and nursing care is directed toward treating disease that results from unhealthy lifestyle behaviors. Activities that prevent disease are designed to promote health, thereby reducing the need for treating and caring for so many sick people. The ministry of the parish nurse can tackle such preventive strategies at the local church level and help people make connections between their physical and mental health and their spiritual wholeness.

Of course, many people engage in their own activities to promote their health. Some read labels on processed foods and avoid foods high in sodium, sugar, and trans fats. Others implement regular exercise routines or attempt various weight loss strategies. Some are intentional about promoting their emotional and mental health by practicing healthy boundaries in their relationships and work lives.

These kinds of health-promoting activities are essential for the PN to emphasize in a church congregation so that the people can prosper in health. The PN partners with the church community to identify areas to target and then to develop programs to promote congregational health. Preventing the development of disease and illness should be a major focus so that the parishioners can model a healthy, God-honoring lifestyle. A reasonable measure of physical and mental wholeness allows Christians to devote more of their time and energy to serving the Lord rather than caring for their illnesses.

Physical Health Programs

Physical health programs at the congregational level will often focus on basic maintenance issues common to all people—namely nutritional eating habits and regular physical exercise to aid weight control and cardiovascular health. Programs may vary depending on the age, starting health, and interests of the congregation.[1]

Nutrition Program

Nina's Baptist church *loved* to eat together—and with so many first-generation immigrants in the congregation who brought their favorite recipes from their country of origin, the food was always amazing! So Nina knew that any health program related to healthy eating would need to balance that vital cultural celebration of flavors and fellowship with a moderate concern for more nutritious options. With that in mind, the PN recruited volunteers from the hospitality committee and from among the best cooks in the church to help with menu planning and program development. She knew that if she could get the cooks on board, the rest of the church would be happy enough to follow.

Dolores was well aware that in her aging congregation, the national trend toward obesity wasn't as much of an issue as unhealthy weight loss among her elderly members. Before she made any plans related to nutrition or exercise, she needed to find out why so many of the church's seniors were dropping pounds that some of them couldn't afford to lose. Soon she discovered a variety of factors at work. Some people complained of joint pain and other mobility issues that made cooking too difficult; others confessed that some months, they had to choose between groceries and their prescription medications; still others shrugged and said that food just didn't taste good anymore, a symptom of advancing age as the senses begin to fail. Dolores knew she would need input and support from an entire team of people to help her address this complex health concern.

Exercise Program
In any health promotion effort, it is helpful to establish a continuum of health to identify where a given individual or group is starting from—and working toward. As goals are achieved, the individual's or group's progress can be marked on that continuum, indicating their advancement toward a healthy balance. A health continuum may be developed for selected health areas relating to physical and mental health.

For example, if a PN wants to develop an exercise program to encourage weight loss and heart health in the congregation, a good starting place would be to develop a continuum for weight status, as follows:

Starvation	Underweight	Recommended Weight	Overweight	Obesity

Activities to promote health should be introduced to help the individual move from the negative to a more positive balance of the continuum. Goals need to be identified and programs initiated to achieve a balanced continuum. For some groups, a tight research study that involves careful observation of food intake might be designed to modify weight. But other times, a less direct approach may be more feasible in order to restore balance for a greater number across the age spectrum. In relation to the categories of *overweight* and *obesity*, a group focus on exercise might be more acceptable to the participants and achieve the same outcome as a designated weight loss program. Persons who are overweight are often very sensitive about this aspect of their health, so a program focusing strictly on weight loss might be unacceptable to some and lead few to participate.

Using the weight scale as a clinical assessment tool in her figurative toolbox, Mary was aware of church members who evidenced a steady gain in weight. They weren't yet showing symptoms of ill health, but if they continued in their current trend, the symptoms of joint pain, knee replacements, heart disease, and other weight-related illnesses were sure to follow. She listened to their comments on food and eating and finally concluded that she needed to approach health promotion for the overweight group by setting up an exercise program. But how to choose one from the variety of options available?

Each exercise program has strengths and weaknesses. As a PN, you will want to choose one that is suitable for your congregation. If the members are largely older adults, look for a program that is sensitive to issues of mobility and reduced energy levels. If most parishioners are parents of young children, a program that can be done across generations might be welcomed for engaging the entire family. If your church is located in a climate not conducive to outdoor activity twelve months a year, consider a program that is focused on indoor activity—or rotate programs with the seasons.

Consider some of these options:

■ National Episcopal Health Ministries offers a website that features a variety of health-related resources for churches (www.episcopalhealth ministries.org). Among those resources is a manual for planning a 5K walk for your congregation, including stretching exercises, a guide for selecting running shoes, and suggestions for advertising and initiating a program. Also featured is a free toolkit for faith communities based on First Lady Michelle Obama's "Let's Move" initiative, which focuses on fighting childhood obesity.

■ "Walk to Jerusalem" is a program in which the PN calculates the total miles from the church building to the city of Jerusalem. Use that total mileage as the goal for your church's exercise program. You will divide that total mileage by the number of participants so that, over a period of time, each participant will walk a leg of the "journey." Once all participants have reached their exercise goal, the accumulated miles walked, run, biked, or swam will have led to the spiritual destination: Jerusalem.

■ "Walk with Our Missionaries" is similar to "Walk to Jerusalem," but it provides your church with a more practical connection with the congregation's mission work. Instead of calculating the distance to Jerusalem, the PN calculates the distance to one or more countries or regions where a church-supported missionary is serving. The mileage or target destination may be adapted for younger or older participants, and the exercise program might also be tied to a fundraiser for a planned mission trip or additional missionary support. Involve the missionaries themselves by telling them about the program and asking them to write messages of encouragement and anecdotes about their missionary work.

Mary really liked the idea of walking with their church-support missionaries. She drafted an Exercise Program Plan that outlined the steps she would need to take to implement this program. (See "Exercise Program Planning" at http://www.judsonpress.com/free_download_book _excerpts.cfm.) In keeping with her program plan, Mary consulted with the healthcare committee to flesh out the idea of figuratively "walking with the missionaries," and then approached the Mission Board to get their support and partnership. Even more thrilling, the deacons volunteered to raise money to award the "top exerciser" (measured in miles or incremental goals met) with an expenses-paid trip to visit the missionary the program had been supporting. Mary knew that was something God's Spirit directed. She silently prayed that the winner might be a young person who could experience mission life first-hand.

Before starting any new exercise program, encourage participants to ask their doctor for guidelines about appropriate activities and weight loss goals. Not all bodies are able to withstand the same level of stress or strain. Most parishioners will need to choose walking over running; some will do better with a recumbent bike than with a spin bike; seniors may require exercise routines done in a straight-back chair, as opposed to lying supine or hustling around the block.

Mental Health Programs

Like physical health programs, programs designed to promote mental health among church members will tend to emphasize issues common to all people—as opposed to highly personal and personalized diagnoses that require referrals to licensed therapists or credentialed psychiatrists. Such programs *might* include support groups centered on grief or addictions, including groups cosponsored with other community organizations. Many twelve-step programs, such as Alcoholics Anonymous, Overeaters Anonymous, and Gamblers Anonymous, meet in churches and welcome members of the community as well as church members to attend. Other programs might address specific concerns with creative ministry responses, such as Parents' Night Out programs that support single parents and give married couples a date night. Programs will vary depending on the identified concerns and the resources of the congregation.

Overcoming Loneliness

Everyone feels lonely sometimes. Some feel lonely in the midst of a throng, such as the parent of young children who is desperate for adult conversation, or the senior living in a crowded nursing home with no family or friends who visit. Others are isolated emotionally, such as the adult with an "empty nest," or the newly widowed or divorced spouse who is at a loss on the social scene. And some are isolated physically, when ill health keeps them confined at home or prevents them from seeing friends or distant family. Some children experience loneliness too, especially when faced with a new school or a new neighborhood.

A continuum can be used to represent a level of social interaction and engagement in activities:

Overcommitted	Limited Time	Balanced Engagement	Loneliness	Isolation

Typically loneliness occurs when an individual's social interaction decreases. For most people, their realm of relationships usually starts with their parents, expanding to include extended family and close friends, and then broadening as school and other social activities increase. But when there is a change in the normal pattern—such as a new parent leaving the professional world to stay at home with a child, a divorce or the death of a spouse, or unemployment or retirement requiring a transition from workplace to home—the loss of social stimuli will affect most people. Personality factors contribute to how this change affects an individual, of course, although not always in predictable ways. An extrovert might feel the loss of interaction more profoundly at first but be better equipped to seek new social interactions, while an introvert may adjust readily to the solitude, only to become lost in it with few skills or little motivation to jump back into the world.

The PN who identifies loneliness as a mental health concern in his or her church community might take time to assess the types of loneliness present. Is it most common among parents of young children? Is it epidemic among the elderly whose spouses and friends are rapidly dying off? Or is it more evident among the fifty- and sixty-something folks who are experiencing retirement or empty nests as their adult children move out and away?

Then the PN might identify the exceptions to the loneliness phenomenon. Which stay-at-home caregivers seem to have vibrant connections with other adults? Which retirees have found new passion for life in travel or a hobby? Which elders are sustaining a lively social life, and with whom? What potential might there be to build relational bridges between the different groups of lonely people within the same church community? For example, would the empty nesters welcome an opportunity to spend an afternoon babysitting for the young parent or perhaps visiting the homebound elderly?

After taking time to investigate who among his church family were lonely, Jake opted to concentrate first on the homebound elderly group. He had received many phone calls from that group, which was powerful testimony to their sense of isolation. In considering his program options, Jake decided against any kind of educational workshop on the topic of loneliness. This health concern seemed to recommend an ongoing program more than a one-time event, and he wanted the program to offer a significant break from the mundane routines of the homebound. They craved meaningful social interaction, and that's what Jake wanted to provide.

After consulting with his healthcare committee, Jake devised two different plans. One was an adopt-an-elder visitation program, in which active parishioners were asked to "match" with one of the homebound members and to commit to visiting that person at least twice a month. He promoted it as a "want ad":

Wanted! Pioneers for a new venture. We need people to make some special visits this year. Will you volunteer? You can crack jokes, play music, tell (and hear) stories, and be an encouragement to some people in our congregation who can no longer get out to church services.

He was delighted when the initial response netted a dozen volunteers who were eager to get started. Some wanted to visit in pairs; a few asked to be matched with specific individuals with whom they had some distant connection. Jake gave the volunteers a brief discussion on topics of practical use in visiting, which together formed an acrostic of the word HOMEBOUND:

H umor (See Humor Notes at http://www.judsonpress.com/free _download_book_excerpts.cfm.)
O bservation of person and environment
M usic
E ncouragement
B askets of faith and fun
O ccupational activities
U nderstanding impaired communication
N utritional issues of concern
D eath and coping

The volunteers seemed grateful to have these ideas as a starting place for their first visits.

The second program Jake designed involved a partnership with the Missions Board, which invited the homebound members to contribute to a mission project. They were asked to knit, carve, crochet, or otherwise create some kind of gift for designated recipients; sometimes the recipients were children in the hospital, and other times they were residents of the home for mentally disabled adults. Other homebound members were asked to contribute notes and cards for birthdays, anniversaries, and get-well messages to other church members. Before long, Jake was hearing from everyone involved about new friendships being formed and a renewed sense of connection between the homebound members and the rest of the congregation.

This chapter targeted nutrition, exercise, and loneliness as special-need areas on which to focus. To promote health in these areas, PNs need to focus on the major factor contributing to the need. For example, nutrition may be over abundant, leading to obesity, or inadequate, leading to extreme weight loss. Loneliness can be all-consuming, affecting physical, mental, and emotional health, so programs may create interaction with other people (visitation) or distraction through other-centered activities (service projects such as letter writing and knitting). Depending on the needs of a given group, the promotion of health must be directed toward achieving a more balanced state. After the PN in conjunction with the congregation targets areas of need, health promoting activities can be directed to these needs.

Questions

1. How might a weight loss program in your church integrate faith?

2. Why might a church support group for weight loss be especially meaningful and helpful?

3. What examples of too little or too much social engagement are evident in your church?

4. How might visiting the homebound people be used to reduce some of their loneliness?

5. What might your church parishioners find hardest about visiting the homebound?

Notes

1. See http://www.healthypeople.gov/2020/topicsobjectives2020/default.aspx and http://www.cdc.gov/nchs/healthy_people/hp2010/hp2010_focus_areas.htm.

CHAPTER 10

Outreach of the Parish Nurse

One minister refused to locate his church in a building at a specific address. When asked where his church was, he paused thoughtfully before listing places where he knew members worked. He believed that the church was not a building, but the sphere of influence members have as they live out their lives reflecting the service mission of their Lord.

Traditionally, churches make efforts to draw people into our places of worship and ministry. Once they are inside the building, we are eager to tell them about Christ's love for them. We see evidence of such ministry when ushers greet visitors, when musicians minister in music, and when teachers lead discussions in classes. Some sermons can be considered outreach because they are seeker-centered and intended to reach those in the pews who are unfamiliar with the gospel; other sermons are designed to equip church members to go out and share Christ's love in their daily life experiences. These latter messages might be deemed disciple-making as opposed to evangelistic.

Ministry programs in the church may be similarly categorized as being geared toward evangelism (reaching *out* to the world and drawing people *in* with the Good News) or discipleship (equipping those already "inside" for the purpose of sending them "outside"). Deacon ministry usually focuses on the pastoral care and spiritual growth of church members (discipleship); the work of the mission's board is usually focused outside the church, serving or supporting ministry in the world as a way to proclaim the gospel in word and deed (evangelism).

In some cases, however, a ministry or vocational role has a dual focus. Parish nursing is such a role. It is very much engaged in ministry to and with church members. As already described, much of the PN's work happens in the church facilities and in regular ministry contexts. But as described, the PN is also called to go out into the community, not only visiting church members in their homes and hospital rooms but also partnering with other faith communities and organizations around health concerns. And any opportunity to leave the church facility is also a chance to carry the model of Christian service and God's love into the world.

In their daily work focused on serving others at points of need, nurses are often given opportunities to meet needs with Christian grace. PNs may plan programs that are attractive to people at a physical health level but that also interface with spiritual health. That isn't to say that PNs will necessarily be involved in typical outreach programs of evangelism and missions work. However, PNs are in frequent contact with the community, and as representatives of the local church they can act as ambassadors of Christ's love in the world, inviting new people into the church environment to interact with others from the congregation and learn more about the Christian faith.

Community Liaison

As a community liaison with members of the professional community, the PN has opportunity to make contacts with many healthcare providers such as physicians, nurses, occupational therapists, physical therapists, and pharmacists, just to name a few. Typically such encounters are brief and not suited to traditional evangelism or the sharing of a personal testimony. However, through commitment to such community collaboration and by evidencing a spirit of Christian compassion and service, the Spirit's fruits—love, joy, peace, patience, kindness, goodness, faithfulness, gentleness, and self-control (Galatians 5:22-23, RSV)—are evident.

Mary spent a number of hours with the local Red Cross group in planning a blood drive using Mountain View Church's Activity Center. She had coordinated volunteers from the congregation who assisted with registration, distributing snacks, and providing childcare for blood donors. Jake had worked with the Chamber of Commerce to establish a first aid station during two local city events. Church members with first aid certification had staffed the station, located just inside the church's side door. Dolores had facilitated the use of church classroom space for local first responders to do CPR training, and through her promotional efforts in the congregation, several church members attended and earned their certificates. Nina had collaborated with the local school district to offer space and volunteers for ESL tutoring. As part of the arrangement, Nina herself had been present to answer questions about healthcare available to new and undocumented immigrants.

At such events, PNs often find that a significant percentage of the participants are from the community. The prayer is that the interactions between PN, church members, and community residents will be positive, mutually rewarding, and a consistently faithful witness to Christian love.

Community Nursing

Community nursing is a blend of key practices used in primary healthcare (accessible general medical and dental care) that are more community-based within the context of health promotion and illness prevention. Such care is often targeted toward population groups (e.g., children, the elderly, the poor) within a community. If the health promotion care is optimum, primary healthcare would be markedly reduced. Community health nurses develop comprehensive health programs that pay special attention to social and ecological concerns and specific at-risk populations. Note that community health nurses are distinguished from home care nurses, who also work in the community but provide specific technical care, such as intravenous administration, to individual persons.

Mary was surprised at how quickly word had spread to the neighboring residents that a nurse was located in the church. Rather than go to an Urgent Care center, some of the neighbors stopped by the church. She tabulated that she had twenty-five visits from local people wondering about their blood pressure, their weight, a child's rash, or other non-emergency concerns like assessment after a fall. She had directed a few to Urgent Care or other sources for assistance. Mary was happy to see that several of the neighbors who came to her had also begun coming to Mountain View for church services.

PNs often collaborate with churches who don't have PNs and with PN colleagues by inviting members of other churches to health programs on topics of interest, such as Alzheimer's prevention, child abuse, and Neighborhood Watch Programs. This collaboration enhances interfaith relationships.

Jake participated in a planning committee meeting with the local Lutheran church's PN. A number of other community members from the local university as well as from the hospital were there to plan for the development of a free clinic. With the economic downturn and so many already homeless people, a lot of people could not afford healthcare insurance. Pastor Sue and the healthcare committee had agreed with Jake to commit their congregation's participation in this clinic work. Jake wanted to help with the planning and then get some of the church members with medical training to participate in the clinic work as well.

Health Fair

Fairs of almost any kind seem to draw crowds. There is a degree of excitement about local county fairs. They usually are a fun-filled summer activity. With well-designed displays and mini demos, they are highly interactive. Health fairs are a good way to highlight healthy activities and to introduce new health behaviors. With effective advertising, community health fairs serve to bring focus to health issues of concern as well as promote ecumenical work.

Themes

Fair themes can be as varied as people. Themes are important in order to appeal to selected community groups and might include nutrition, men's or women's health, or older adult health. A fair with the theme of school health, for example, might feature immunizations, dental checks, and vision screening. It might also present topics of interest such as school lunch health and stocking vending machines. Most students are fascinated by police cars, school buses, and fire trucks, so tours of these vehicles would provide plenty of enjoyment. Games could offer winners book binders, lunch kits (if these are used by children in the area), toothbrushes and toothpaste, and special soaps. Whatever the chosen theme, the whole fair can be organized around it.

Food

Refreshments and nutrition are another key focus that lends itself well to a fair experience. Traditional snacks such as cotton candy, sugary drinks, and caramel apples can be swapped for healthy alternatives. For instance, bananas covered in peanut butter could be offered instead of deep-fried watermelon sticks. Nutritionists might provide helpful suggestions for snack and lunch items.

Parish nurse Pattie Boyes has provided simple guidelines for a church health fair emphasizing the point that it should be fun—conducted as a party.[1] Boyes organized her material using a key nursing tool, often called the nursing process (assessment, planning, implementation, and evaluation). Boyes asked simple questions to assess the need for and planning for a fair: "Who will benefit?" and "Who will help?" Under implementation she described setting up tables, chairs, signs, and equipment the night before so that on the day of the fair she could relax and greet guests. With respect to evaluation she queried exhibitors, speakers, and visitors. For the longer-term evaluation she asked, "What impact did the health fair have?" in areas related to exercise and nutrition.

Common wisdom holds that health fairs should raise health awareness and provide educational experiences and materials. Consider providing a lot of take-away items, including printed materials and samples such as sunblock, toothbrushes, toothpaste, soap, hand sanitizer, and mouthwash. Because a health fair is also an outreach opportunity, the church may want to give away items imprinted with the church's contact information, such as ink pens, notepads, string bags, or water bottles.

While a health fair can consist primarily of static displays that offer photos or diagrams as illustrations, real demonstrations will be more engaging and interactive. For example, one exhibit might feature a demonstration of flossing teeth on a plastic denture model, while another booth could offer participants the opportunity to practice thorough hand-washing while humming the "Happy Birthday" song through twice. Small classrooms, as opposed to one large common area, may offer greater privacy for more personalized demos, such as blood sugar monitoring or body mass index calculation. Other demonstrations might include interactions related to nutrition, exercise, stress management, ergonomic work space and habits, and more.

Time and Date

A lot of factors need to be considered in scheduling a major event like a health fair: weather, church and community calendars, guest speakers' schedules, health awareness months, and so on. The congregational culture and demographics need to be considered as well. If most church members are retired and dislike driving at night, a midweek fair from 8:00 a.m. to 4:00 p.m. or 12:00 p.m. to 3:00 p.m. might work well, but if many have day jobs, then evenings or weekends are the times to use. If the target audience is children and youth and their parents, a summer event while kids are out of school may be best. If a number of church members live outside the church's immediate neighborhood (commuter church members), planning the fair for Sunday afternoon might ease the burden of a second commute and raise the attendance.

Purpose behind Activities and Exhibits

Fair organizers need to determine the purpose for holding the fair, and then they can decide which activities and exhibits would best relate to the purpose. Selecting proper activities and program events is key to planning a good fair. Games and fun for all participants should be a given.

If the fair is of a general health nature, children, adults, and seniors could be brought together in intergenerational activities to learn about different health approaches selected at different times in life. Question-and-answer sessions would be useful particularly related to educational topics that might be controversial, such as mandating immunizations for children and older adults. An educational discussion of the pros and cons of preventing a disease such as shingles would support this general purpose. Similarly, following a presentation on the illness outcome of corn syrup, a question and answer session would expand thinking and hopefully convince some to reduce intake of foods containing high amounts of this sugar.

Health Fair Planning in Action

A health fair may be the most complex and time-consuming program a PN undertakes, especially if the goal includes community outreach and ecumenical or interfaith collaboration. The more partners an event involves, the more details and human beings to coordinate. That need not discourage the motivated PN, but it should alert one to the need for advance planning (See Appendix G).

In addition to the factors noted above, consider these details:

- Program goals (informational, educational, interactive, entertaining)
- Budget
- Volunteers
- Community sponsors or partners

■ Registration (when to do it; what information to collect)

■ Intergenerational considerations (activities for the very young or very old; accessibility for those with special needs; childcare)

■ Program content (classes, activities, exhibits; see Figure 5 below for ideas)

■ Resources for sale and purchase

■ Items for giveaway

■ Refreshments (free, by donation, or priced)

■ Promotion and advertising of event

■ Exhibit and vendor space (free or for a fee; invitation-only or open to community)

Figure 5/ Ideas for Health Fair Classes, Activities, and Exhibits

Physical	Mental	Spiritual
Exercise class	Alzheimer's prevention	Christian meditation class
Body Mass Index calculation	Computer blocking	
Low carbohydrate class	Reading club	Bible stories
Dental screening	Counselors:	Spiritual direction
Hearing screening	• marriage	Sample Bible study class
Vision screening	• substance abuse	
Blood pressure screening	Support Groups:	Word Study Tool class
Blood cholesterol calculation	• Stop smoking	
Life span health	• AA, Al-Anon	Homebound visiting
Breast and testicular self- exam —plastic model demo	Depression screening	Unceasing prayer— discussion
	Encouragement class	Pastor—questions on faith
Doctor—questions	Humor gallery	
Pharmacist—questions	Psychologist Q&A	Resources for Christian families
Health lifeline	Stress-management talks	Gideon booth—Bibles

Consider developing a task force model for addressing some of these bigger concerns, such as one team of volunteers focused on soliciting vendors to rent exhibit space while another group works on promoting the event itself through local media outlets and with other community organizations and faith communities.

Post-Event Evaluation

Finally, don't neglect to plan for follow-up. How will you assess the effectiveness and success of the event? One option is a brief written survey form, perhaps with the incentive of attendees being eligible for a prize drawing if they complete and submit the survey before leaving the event. If e-mails or other contact information are collected from attendees as part of registration, a brief online survey might net reasonable response rates. Of course, collecting anecdotal feedback from church members who volunteered or participated will also be valuable input.

Get feedback from the planning team as well. Meet soon after the event to debrief. What worked and what didn't work? Was attendance better or worse than expected? Did the event stay within budget or exceed it—and if the latter, in what areas? What supplies ran out and which items are still around in quantity? Which vendors seemed to be well received? Which exhibits had the most traffic, and which had the least? Overall, was the event worth the time, effort, and energy expended?

Be sure to ask around about community feedback as well. Were there any complaints from the neighbors about noise, traffic, or litter? Did residents come out to see what was happening? Among those community members who did attend, how did they learn about the event and what was the main attraction for their participation?

Grief Support

Death, often more frequent than new babies and new marriages, is a part of the rhythm of life in any faith community. Some years will seem to be nearly overwhelmed by grief, including the passing of longtime and beloved elders of the church and sometimes the tragic or traumatic loss of a child or spouse who dies "too soon." Long after the funeral or memorial service is over, the parish church nurse may be sensitive to the lingering waves of grief. Visitation with family members and touching base with close friends of the deceased are vital parts of PN ministry. But in those seasons when death seems to be a constant companion and grief hangs like a low, dark shadow over the congregation, a different, more holistic approach such as grief support is needed.

After attending eight funerals in the past year, Nina saw that her top priority as PN at First Spanish Baptist Church was to set up a grief support class. While she would certainly connect with the eight recently bereaved families to invite their participation, Nina knew that even (and sometimes especially) people who were struggling under the burden of long-standing grief would benefit from this new ministry program.

It was not very hard to identify the purpose: *Conduct a support group to share the comfort of God when an individual has experienced some form of loss.* Outlining her objectives took Nina a little more time, but the final list was as follows:

1. Define selected terms such as *loss*, *grief*, and *grief recovery*.
2. Identify the grief patterns described by experts in the field.
3. Describe grief behaviors, feelings, and spiritual questions and concerns.
4. Discuss activities that help externalize some of the pain of grief.
5. Practice using some coping approaches that aid in dealing with grief. (See "Coping Approaches" at http://www.judsonpress.com/ free_download_book_excerpts.cfm.)
6. Look for signs of your own healing with respect to your grief experience.

Nina decided on a six-week time frame for the grief support class. (See "Sample Grief Support Sessions" at www.judsonpress.com/free_down

load_book_excerpts.cfm.) She knew that recovery from a profound grief experience did not occur rapidly. She talked with several of the people she hoped would participate to find out the best time for them to attend. Then she prepared a flyer to promote the class in the neighborhood and an announcement for the local newspaper and church bulletin. (See "Grief Support Announvement" at http://www.judsonpress.com/free_download_book_excerpts.cfm.)

When the PN invites community people to participate in a grief support program, the implicit message is that the church cares about them when they are struggling with their grief. The PN's outreach potential, by offering a community grief support invitation, is profound.

As people come to the church, their presence offers an opportunity to introduce them to the care and love of Christ. Health fairs focus on health just as our Lord did as part of his earthly ministry. Jesus was concerned about food for the multitudes (Matthew 14:19-20) and reducing stress for his disciples (Matthew 14:22). Among the many people he healed, Jesus opened the eyes of a blind man lying beside the road (John 9:1).

A grief support program serves to open spiritual eyes. Jesus came to Mary and Martha to care for them in their grief over the death of their brother Lazarus. A grief support program does not bring the dead person back to life as Jesus raised Lazarus, but it does provide comfort for those in grief who often may be struggling with physical, emotional, and spiritual symptoms accompanying their loss. Reaching out to people who are dealing with loss eventually assists them in turning to life again. For those who have no church home, such comfort and encouragement truly draws them into church and, if they are not believers, may also serve to draw them to the Lord.

PNs initiate programs and make individual contacts that provide a way to bring people to the church building through events such as health fairs and grief support groups. A grief support program is primarily an individual outreach, while the health fair extends to many. The PN also has an opportunity to reach other health professionals by enlisting their support in sponsoring a community health fair. Contacts through these activities afford opportunities to demonstrate Christian living in action.

Questions

1. How might a PN reach out to the community around your church?

2. What services draw people living around your church building to step inside?

3. What kinds of programs might PNs in churches around yours work on cooperatively?

4. What are some ways the promotion of health can become fun?

5. While experiencing grief, people are especially sensitive. How might a PN build bridges for people from the community to come to the church for comfort?

6. What resources does a church offer for reaching out to a grieving community?

Notes

1. Pattie Boyes, "Church Health Fairs: Partying with a Purpose," *Journal of Christian Nursing* 18 (Summer 2001): 17–19.

CHAPTER 11

Variations in Parish Nursing

When you step into the PN role, it takes a little time to realize that different churches and other groups have developed their PN positions in different ways and even with different names (see Chapter 2). One church might have a model that requires one PN for that church, while two other churches might have a model that allows them to share one PN between them. Some PNs are paid staff (like Mary) and others are volunteers. Even the scope of a PN's activities or the way programs are initiated may vary.

Networking with other PNs and churches at local and national levels provides a helpful perspective on some of the diversities. Church funds designated for continuing PN education may allow for a PN to travel to special programs that offer more background on the development and expansion of parish nursing, not to mention opportunities for dialogue among PN colleagues. The annual Westberg Symposium, now sponsored by the Church Health Center (www.parishnurses.org), is a great choice for parish nurses who are eager to network with their peers and learn more about trends and issues in the vocation. The symposium honors the pioneering work of Granger Westberg, recognized as the founder of parish nursing. PNs who enjoy continuing education benefits as members of their church staff can use those CE dollars toward registration, travel, and accommodations.

Models-Practice Variations

Different sources propose various models for parish nursing. The four models described by Jane Simington, Joanne Olson, and Lillian Douglass in their 1966 article on parish nursing remain the predominant practices across the vocation.[1]

Community Health or Hospital-Based Model

This type of parish nursing program is administered by a community group or a hospital. Local churches or groups agree to sponsor a nurse to participate in this type of program. As an example, Jo Ann Gragnani[2] was hired in 1986 by the Missionary Sisters of the Sacred Heart of Jesus, who operate Cabrini Medical Center in an inner-city community of Chicago. Gragnani described her work as "case management" and made home visits and consulted with hospitals and clinics. She regularly took blood pressure readings and initiated nutrition education programs.

Parish-Directed Model

A nurse is hired by a church or other faith community to offer health promotion and preventive services. Most of the examples described in this volume feature PNs in this model, including Mary's position at Mountain View Church.

Regional Parish Nursing Model

In this model, parish nurse work is directed by a regional board, synod (ecclesiastical council), or diocese (sphere of church authority). Of the three, the regional body makes decisions about programming. In a given region the programs are the same, unless the regional group directs that changes be made for the special needs of a given parish due to demographics or other factors.

Terri was hired by a synod and was responsible for implementing the programs the synod had designated based on their view of current health needs. In reviewing demographics of the churches in this synod, she found that most of the congregational members were middle-aged and older. So she recommended programs relevant to the needs of members in this age group, such as:

1. Mild exercise
2. Alzheimer's disease prevention
3. Caregiver training
4. Caregiver respite
5. Decision-making for living facilities based on chronic illnesses

Terri was responsible for developing the programs with assistance from resource people, and then she organized presentation logistics such as time, place, and advertising. Terri, along with experts in each area, implemented the programs and then evaluated each program based on participants' experiences and their ratings of program objectives.

Coalition Model
In a coalition model, various church denominations, social organizations, and health and educational institutions collaborate to provide a parish nursing network, to which different groups subscribe for specific services and program assistance.

Dan was hired by a coalition of area churches, a community hospital, and a community college. The coalition identified specific services and programs that they could offer to the members of these groups. Some of the services included the following:

1. Prayer with individuals in churches, hospitals, or schools
2. Assessment of a given local group to identify their needs
3. Health assessment clinics that discuss blood pressure, weight, and nutrition
4. Exercise programs for selected groups such as the disabled, frail, or ill

5. Programs focused on one's spiritual journey toward health and wholeness

Variations in Initiating a PN Program

A PN program typically starts when individuals or groups of people sense a need to promote health in a way that includes spiritual aspects of faith traditions. Westberg was a Lutheran chaplain, so the initial programs he founded originated in this Christian faith tradition. But a number of other religious and secular groups may also choose to introduce spiritual dimensions of health.

A ministerial association gives pastors the opportunity to connect with other pastors as they discuss the health needs arising in their congregations. One pastor may describe an article he read about parish nursing, and another may tell about a church with a successful PN program.

Nurses who read literature about parish nursing become interested in what a PN does. As they assess needs in their church congregation, they may think about volunteering to help with some health-related activities. Sometimes community nurses become particularly interested because they see a direct relationship between their secular work and what might be done in their local church community to promote health in the body of Christ.

Smaller hospitals, sometimes those without chaplains, decide to explore the role a PN might take in their institution. Community service groups decide to assist with some of the religious/spiritual needs they identify in their clients. Colleges and universities, especially those with nursing programs, may want to engage a PN to teach about the integration of faith and health.

Mary was delighted to encounter her PN friend, Dolores, at this year's Westberg Symposium, and Dolores introduced her to three other PN colleagues, Nina, Pat, and Jake. They met for lunch and the conversation turned to how each nurse's local church had started a PN ministry.

"My church is located in the suburbs," Pat said, to get the ball rolling. "If we were closer to a major city, we would have a Wholistic Health Center like Westberg's fifty years ago. In the 'burbs, we have a lot of clinics and services of all kinds. But our congregation is concerned about the needs of the hidden people in our community—the homeless and those with low incomes who can't afford healthcare. The idea of a parish nurse program came out of the Missions Board, which was always highlighting the needs of the homeless. One of the elders, a friend, knew I was an RN with a specialization in community nursing. The church leaders invited me to come in and talk to them about what was involved. A few months later, they had crafted a job description and offered me the opportunity to come on staff and establish the PN program. I jumped at the chance. Working on promoting the health of people who have not been very healthy is satisfying." Pat paused. "I feel like a true Good Samaritan every day. When asked why I'm there, I can truly say, 'I am here to serve you in the name of Jesus.'"

"Well, no one asked me to be a PN, and I don't get paid anything. I just began," Nina admitted. "We have a lot of undocumented immigrants in our congregation, and many of them are afraid to seek traditional medical care. So when I saw the need, especially among the children and elders in our church, I told the pastor what I wanted to do and just put out my shingle. I started with setting up a blood pressure assessment in a corner of the church lobby one Sunday. I told people that I was a licensed nurse and that I wanted to share my health and medical knowledge with them. Word spread through the church and community grapevine, and now people from the neighborhood are coming to me too."

"If you initiate a program on a volunteer basis, it is easier to get going quickly. Then you don't need a line item in the budget and have to wait for all that to be voted on and cleared," Dolores agreed. "I am paid now, but initially I just started doing things. I even set up a talk line for the caregivers. We have a lot of seniors and typically one cares for the other.

Lots of them have worries and concerns that can be handled by a few minutes of my time on the phone, or talking with another seasoned caregiver. I had been doing the volunteer work for about three months when one of the church elders came to me telling me how much my work was appreciated. He said they were adding a budget line to pay me for twenty hours a week to work as a PN." Dolores shook her head. "You could have knocked me over with a feather. I hadn't realized people really noticed what I was doing."

Jake chimed in, describing a different way to initiate a program. "I went the long way around. Having grown up in my church, I knew our congregation liked to have things well-planned. So after I graduated from nursing school, I put together a job description and submitted it to the church board. They called me in to ask some questions about exactly what they might expect to have me do. They were keen to follow Christ's example and establish a healing ministry. I focused on some of the things that would improve health—an exercise program, nutrition education, and so on. The board finally designated funds for three days a week. Obviously, I can't do as much in three days as I'd like to do. I sometimes put in extra hours, which I just consider my ministry role," Jake admitted.

Jake's friend Dan had joined their lunch group, and he spoke up now. "You have all been talking about church-based PN programs. I was a business major before I became a nurse, so it seemed normal for me to think about groups and businesses. When I first learned about parish nursing, I wanted to merge it with my interest in business. I contacted hospitals, the local community college, and my own church leadership. Now we have formed a coalition—I can provide healthcare *and* work with different institutions. And I even get paid!" he grinned.

Terri was a former classmate of Dolores's from nursing school. "My experience was different from any of yours. I got excited about faith community nursing and really wanted to get into it, but my own parish is small. I would not have had enough work to do. So I contacted our area diocese. The leaders immediately bought in. Even the younger priests thought promoting health was essential—look at all the Catholic hospitals there are. So I started to develop programs and present them in different churches, as well as in some of the Catholic hospitals."

Cost of PN Program

As illustrated in the anecdotes above, the idea of a parish nurse ministry is exciting and valued in many congregations. The concern is how to fund it. Most churches want to pay their PN for the critical services being offered, but how can they work it into the already strained church budget? Before initiating a parish nurse program, it is important for a church to count the costs of some basic essentials. Some of those expense items are identified as follows:[3]

- Office space
- Computer or tablet and cell phone
- Supplies, including postage and paper
- Parish nurse basic nursing curriculum ($500 to $1,500 online; see Chapter 2 for typical content)
- Salary (part-time or full-time)
- Continuing education
- Benefits, including healthcare insurance

These costs are sobering when considering the introduction of a PN program. This is why some churches have decided to share one PN. Others have paid for only part-time employment. Some groups have found that the idea of a phase-in program works out well, wherein the ministry is established on a shoestring budget of only a few thousand dollars. Then, as the program grows and the church and community come to value the PN's services, additional funds for salary, benefits, and continuing education can be added. (However, note that the full-time PN with benefits is a rare position in the vocation. Most PNs are part-time and many are volunteers.)

Funding for a new parish nurse ministry may come from various sources, not limited to the traditional line item in the church's general or mission budget. Some congregations hold regular fundraisers, such as auctions, car washes, dinners, or walks, to support a salaried PN. Others request monetary donations from interested church members or from denominational and community supporters. Some churches write grants and apply for funding from foundations. And in some cases, individual donors will step forward with memorial gifts or endowments in honor of a loved one who benefited from the PN's ministry during a final illness.

Church Receptivity to Parish Nurse Ministry

As with most new ideas, opinions will vary as to the usefulness and acceptability of the proposed innovation. Even the introduction of the light bulb brought different opinions as to its safety, practicality, and cost. Similarly, parish nursing has strong advocates as well as naysayers.

Those who reject parish nursing often say that their church focus is mission and evangelism, not healthcare. Pastors usually agree that following Christ's model requires ministering to physical needs—but they may not rank such physical ministry as equal in priority with the "spiritual" work of the Great Commission. Therefore, adding a parish nurse ministry to the church's programs and budget may be seen as taking away from the "core" mission of the church. In this situation a volunteer PN might be acceptable if no funds would be diverted. Health promotion programs could then be introduced to illustrate how healthy parishioners can serve in mission work and all other church endeavors more effectively.

Some churches resist developing a PN program because they believe it will interfere with the work of the pastors—especially with the pastoral care relationship with seniors and homebound members. A clear job description and list of activities for the PN can ensure that there will be no overlap. Establishment of a health committee will allow the PN to review any changes in the ministry portfolio with the committee, and the committee can address any emerging questions regarding the separation of pastoral and nursing activities.

A few churches may hold that nurses, specifically female nurses, should not be in leadership roles, especially ones that encompass some degree of spiritual care and development. In such church traditions, narrowing the PN's focus to physical and mental health issues may alleviate this concern about gender roles in the church.

A Concluding Word

Ecclesiastes 3:1-8 (NIV) lists a majority of the human life experiences that parish nurses confront in their world of work:

There is a time for everything, and a season for every activity under the heavens:
- a time to be born and a time to die,
- a time to plant and a time to uproot,
- a time to kill and a time to heal,
- a time to tear down and a time to build,
- a time to weep and a time to laugh,
- a time to mourn and a time to dance,
- a time to scatter stones and a time to gather them,
- a time to embrace and a time to refrain from embracing,
- a time to search and a time to give up,
- a time to keep and a time to throw away,
- a time to tear and a time to mend,
- a time to be silent and a time to speak,
- a time to love and a time to hate,
- a time for war and a time for peace.

As a PN, I would add one more season to the list:
A time to learn about health and a time to develop a healthy lifestyle.

The Teacher in Ecclesiastes also indicates that people should enjoy life, eat and drink, and find pleasure in their work (see 3:12-13). In one sense this is what parish nursing is about. The ministry of health promotion encompasses all of life's experiences. The goal is to relate one's faith to life. Parish nursing aims to facilitate the connection between one's health and faith.

It is my prayer that this book will help churches and faith communities to learn about parish nursing in an ideal context and how it serves to integrate the faith and health of their members. And for any nurses who become parish nurses, I am asking God to enable you to use the ideas presented in these chapters to educate and promote the health of your group so that they may be healthy "living stones" brought together to serve the Lord, proclaiming his praises (1 Peter 2:5-9).

Questions

1. Which PN model would be the most useful in your church?

2. How would you begin if you wanted to initiate a PN ministry in your church?

3. How would you vary a PN position so that it would fit into your church?

4. How might your church raise money for a PN ministry?

5. How could a volunteer PN position be useful?

6. Do you think a PN would be accepted in your church? Why or why not?

7. How might the activities of the PN be changed to make the position more acceptable in your church?

Notes

1. Jane Simington, Joanne Olson, and Lillian Douglass, "Promoting Well-Being within a Parish," *The Canadian Nurse* 92 (January 1966): 20–24.

2. Jo Ann Gragnani, "Parish Nurse Ministry," *Health and Development* 9, no. 2 (1989): 16–19.

3. Deborah Patterson, *The Essential Parish Nurse: ABCs for Congregational Health Ministry,* (Cleveland, OH: The Pilgrim Press, 2003), 125–129.

Congregational Healthcare Committee

Purpose
Focus on the integration of faith, beliefs, and values with concern for normal, predictable life cycle changes that impact health for the EBC community.

Goals
- Identify healthcare needs according to developmental stages of the EBC community.
- Plan programs, bulletin boards, and other special events to facilitate faith integration related to health needs.
- Evaluate effects of faith and health-related ministry within the EBC community.
- Plan faith and health events that offer outreach opportunity to the surrounding church community and other persons representing all phases of the lifespan.

Through careful planning by the Healthcare Committee it is hoped that personal health concerns and related social service concerns and needs will be addressed within our church setting. Through presenting educational programs, organizing support groups, providing counsel on specific healthcare problems, and coordinating and training volunteers for specific service ministry roles we hope to provide for the health needs within our congregation.

James (2:14-26) urges us to show our faith by the way we live our lives. Church ministry through activities planned by our Healthcare Committee provides a meaningful way to put our faith into action by meeting faith and health-related needs existing within our body of believers.

Activity Examples
1. Offer health-related programs—usually two each year
2. Offer grief recovery programs
3. Arrange travel for those wanting specific social activities
4. Visit of homebound persons unable to attend church service
5. Initiate 90's Club
6. Set up special training programs such as CPR
7. Identify guidelines for ushers and healthcare personnel for medical emergencies
8. Offer blood pressure assessment

Source: E.B.C. Healthcare Committee
Date reviewed: September 2013.

Congregational Health Assessment

Please respond to all items to the best of your ability.

Demographics: Please check appropriate blank or add specific numbers requested.

_____ Male _____ Female

_____ Age

_____ Number of Dependents in Household _____ Ages

_____ Marital Status

_____ Educational Experience

_____ Employed _____ Student _____ Retired

_____ Church Attendance _____ Weekly _____ Other

General Health Status: For each item, check the column that best describes your status.

	Excellent	Good	Poor
General health			
Eating habits			
Exercise routine			
Sleep pattern			
Dental practices			
Ability to cope with stress			
Living accommodations			
Memory			
Problem-solving skills			
Creative thinking ability			
Spiritual well-being			
Emotional well-being			
Interpersonal relationships			
Communication skills			
Other:			

Briefly respond to each of the next four items in the box provided.

Belief and Meaning What gives meaning and purpose to your life?	
Rituals and Practices What are your usual religious rituals that provide structure for your life?	
Courage and Growth How courageous or hopeful are you? Please check one: _____ Very _____ Somewhat _____ Not at all	
Authority and Guidance Where do you find authority for your life? Please check all that apply: _____ Scripture _____ Religious beliefs and teachings _____ Friends and family _____ Other	

Identification of Learning Needs

Please check all that apply:

___ Magazines	___ Doctor	___ Friends
___ Books	___ Nurse	___ Family
___ Internet	___ TV	

Number your top four learning interests (1, 2, 3, 4), with "1" being the highest priority:

___ Exercise

___ Nutrition

___ Relaxation

___ Parenting skills

___ Time management training

___ Quitting smoking

___ Drug and alcohol addictions

___ Abuse: physical, sexual, emotional, financial

___ Aging process

___ Retirement planning

___ Advance directives/ living wills

___ First aid/CPR

___ Men's health

___ Women's health

___ Marriage enrichment

___ Babysitter training

___ Spiritual healing

___ Prayer and fasting

___ Disease information (specify which disease: _____)

___ Stress management

___ Anger management

___ Conflict resolution

___ Coping with depression and loneliness

___ Medication management

___ Sex education

___ Infertility

___ Menopause

___ Miscarriage: support and healing

___ Pre- and postnatal teaching

___ Dealing with homosexuality

___ Caregiving skills

___ Death/dying; grief and loss

___ Medical ethics (e.g., organ donation)

___ Family budgeting

___ Spiritual maturity

___ Spiritual meditation

___ Contentment

Other: _____

Need and Asset Inventory

Indicate the areas in which you need help, and those in which you can offer help.

I Need

___ Transportation assistance
___ Shopping assistance
___ Home visit
___ Prayer support
___ Healthcare information

___ Writing will/setting up trust

___ Housekeeping assistance
___ Caregiving assistance
___ Telephone contact
___ Medical form completion

___ Support group
___ Power of attorney help
___ Advance directive explanation
___ Community resource information
___ Personal care assistance

I Can Help

___ Provide transportation
___ Assist with shopping
___ Visit homebound
___ Pray for needs
___ Provide healthcare information

___ Assist with writing will or preparing trust

___ Assist with housekeeping
___ Assist with caregiving
___ Provide telephone contact
___ Assist completing medical form

___ Organize support group
___ Set up power of attorney
___ Explain advance directives
___ Connect with community resources
___ Assist with personal care (hair, nails, foot care)

Name _____

Phone _____

Address _____

(If you prefer anonymity, return this sheet separately from the rest of the questionnaire.)

Priority Learning Needs Identified by Age

Ages 0–19 10 Questionnaires Returned	Ages 20–29 15 Questionnaires Returned	Ages 30–39 25 Questionnaires Returned	Ages 40–49 35 Questionnaires Returned
Primary • Exercise • Nutrition • Drug/alcohol addiction **Secondary** • Abuse • First aid/CPR • Women's health • Post-abortion support & healing • Faith and trust	**Primary** • Spiritual maturity • Nutrition Stress management • Exercise **Secondary** • First aid/CPR • Prayer • Budgeting • Marriage enrichment	**Primary** • Marriage enrichment • Exercise Stress management • Scriptural meditation **Secondary** • Nutrition • Conflict resolution • Faith and trust	**Primary** • Marriage • Enrichment • Retirement planning • Stress management • Spiritual maturity **Secondary** • Relaxation • Prayer • Anger management • Conflict resolution

Ages 50–59 35 Questionnaires Returned	Ages 60–69 15 Questionnaires Returned	Ages 70+ 15 Questionnaires Returned
Primary · Exercise · Marriage enrichment · Time management · Retirement planning · Stress management · Conflict resolution **Secondary** · Relaxation · Prayer · Fasting · Menopause · Caregiving skills · Spiritual maturity · Christian service	**Primary** · Exercise · Nutrition · Marriage enrichment · Aging process · Retirement planning · Prayer · Stress management · Scriptural meditation · Spiritual maturity · Christian service · Faith and trust **Secondary** · Relaxation · Time Management · Budgeting · Spiritual Healing · Fasting · Conflict resolution · Death and dying · Medical ethics · Contentment	**Primary** · Exercise · Aging process **Secondary** · No Response

One-Year Health Plan for Mountain View Church

Month	Health Focus	Resource Person	Learning Approach or Activity
January	Stress Management	Psychologist	Workshop with relaxation practice
	Smoking Reduction	Public Health Dept.	Alternate behaviors; bulletin flyer insert
February	Exercise	Exercise Physiologist	Workshop with handouts describing exercise workout levels
	Heart Month	Physician or other specialist describing heart attack and stroke treatment	Discussion that differentiates heart attack from stroke
March	Aerobic Exercise	Fitness Trainer	Group practice in aerobic exercise by age and strength; "Walk to Jerusalem"
	Nutrition Month	Nutritionist	Lectures and handouts on low-cholesterol lunches; low-sugar snacks
April	Prayer	Pastors	Discussion on types of prayers
	Cancer Month	Researchers	Presentation on cancer research
May	Depression	Psychologist	Techniques for managing depression
	Speech and Hearing	Audiologist	Hearing Testing

Month	Health Focus	Resource Person	Learning Approach or Activity
June	First Aid/CPR	Red Cross First Aid Trainer	Presentation; CPR Practice
	Water Safety Month	Lifeguard	DVD on water safety
July	Christian Meditation	Pastor	Discussion
	Sun Proctection	Parish Nurse	Education
August	Spiritual Maturity for Older Adults	Pastor	Discussion/Panel
	R&R	Time Management Expert	Discussion of ways to carve out personal and family time
September	Solid Spiritual Food	Pastoral Team	Bible Studies
	Immunization Month	Public Health Dept.	Immunization clinic
October	Grief Support	Parish Nurse	Group discussion
	Marriage Enrichment	Panel	Age group talks
November	Child Health	Teachers	Holiday planning discussions
	Alcohol	Alcohol/Drug Representative	Discussion led by person who has overcome addiction
December	Holiday Joy	Family or persons who do something unusual	Multigenerational persons who can share approaches used in previous decades
	Program Evaluation	PN and Staff	Discussions with Healthcare Team to plan programs for subsequent years

Guidelines for Medical Emergencies

Responsibilities for ushers and related healthcare personnel:

1. Provide or direct others to emergency resources in the event of a medical emergency occurring during church services.

2. Assist *trained* rescuers in an emergency.

Usher Responsibilities:

At site of emergency:

1. Identify the emergency.

2. Charge (head) usher determines whether to call 9-1-1* if any of the following responses of the victim apply:

    a. unresponsive to gentle nudging or verbal cues

    b. unable to breathe or having difficulty breathing

    c. choking

    d. suspected heart attack (complaints of chest pain)

    e. suspected stroke (difficulty moving, lopsided facial
       features, slurred speech)

    f. acute allergic response

    g. seizure when victim has no history of seizure lasting longer
       than 5 minutes

    h. continuous, uncontrolled bleeding

    i. head, neck, or back injury *(do not move victim)*

    j. severe vomiting

    k. severe burns

3. Direct someone to call 9-1-1* and go to the door to wave as the ambulance arrives.

4. Know where the wheelchair and first aid boxes are located** and what is in the first aid box.

5. Give no medications.

Crowd control:

1. Have victim lie on pew bench or floor.

2. Reseat people on that bench or nearby area.

3. Notify victim's family members, whether they are at church or at home.

Inform the pastor:

1. Notify the pastor via verbal comment, hand signal, or written note given to someone nearby to deliver.

2. Indicate whether 9-1-1 was called and whether the pastor should end the service or direct the congregation to
    a. Pray,
    b. Sing hymn, or
    c. Leave sanctuary or other room by exit not used by
       emergency personnel.

Note: Charge usher should have CPR training, as he or she may need to initiate CPR before ambulance arrives.

*List the church address and nearest cross streets next to every phone.
**For example, in foyer, in kitchen cupboard.

Revised April 2014 (Review at designated period of time)

Stress Management Workshop Evaluation

1. How would you summarize the key lesson?

_____

_____

_____

_____

2. Which of the techniques described is most suitable for you to use?

_____

_____

_____

3. Why would you choose the technique you indicated in question 2?

_____

_____

_____

_____

Suggestions for the speaker:
_____ No changes—Excellent job!
_____ Provide more examples
_____ Illustrate use of each example in a setting
_____ Reduce time
_____ Other _____

Workshop Details
Circle letter of choice: A = Good; B = OK; C = Needs change
Timing A B C
Describe suggested changes:

_____

_____

Food   A B C
Describe suggested changes:

_____

_____

Room   A B C
Describe suggested changes:

_____

_____

Other   A B C
Describe suggested changes:

_____

_____

Suggestions for other workshops:

_____

_____

_____

_____

_____

_____

Thank you for completing the evaluation. Please return it to the box provided.

Projected Plans for Health Fair

Purpose: Invite church congregations and people from the surrounding community areas to a Health Fair as a community outreach event.

1. Focus on fun in developing greater awareness of particular health-care problems. Learning does not have to be tedious and boring; it can occur in private or with friends. Sometimes we need support in dealing with problems.

2. Provide for health promotion activities of body, mind, and spirit. Include selections in each area.

3. Through areas included, illustrate the personal journey to whole-ness of body, mind, and spirit. People need to choose what to do at the fair.

4. Provide a happy, fun-filled atmosphere in which people are invited to learn more about the interrelationship of physical and spiritual health in personal well-being. Christians don't always just sit in church!

The goals or objectives were further clarified by the following points:

A. We would like to offer a general health fair rather than a cardiac-specific one.

B. We think the design of Mountain View facilities and parking lots accommodate a health fair.

C. We have drafted a tentative list of classes, activities, and exhibits. Are there other areas that need to be included? Any resource people to consider?

D. Should resource materials be strictly Christian in nature, or should they include general information sources? Can exhibitors be asked to provide funds for snacks and other items?

E. Food should include healthy snacks and lunch (turkey dogs). Should food be free or available for a requested donation?

F. Whom should we ask to help with the fair logistics?

G. Identify the date and time for the fair.

H. Request feedback from all participants, whether upon exiting or via follow-up e-mail. Craft an evaluation based on the program goals (see Chapter 10). Be sure to ask respondents to indicate their involvement (e.g., attendee, presenter, exhibitor, volunteer).

Pastoral Vocation Resources

Ministry can take many more shapes than serving as solo pastor of a local church. If you're exploring or reconsidering your pastoral vocation, add these volumes to your library! Each title is part of Judson's best-selling "Work of the Church" series.

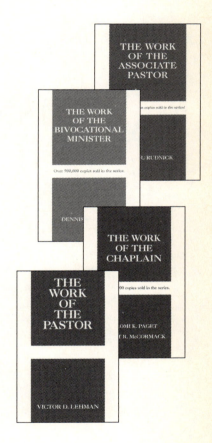

The Work of the Parish Church Nurse is the latest addition to the best-selling "Work of the Church" series.

With more than 1 million copies sold in the series, it's in good company!

AVAILABLE "WORK OF" TITLES INCLUDE:

The Church Business Meeting R. Dale Merrill 978-0-8170-0409-5 $10.00

Work of the Church David R. Sawyer 978-0-8170-1116-1 $10.00

The Work of the Church Officers Glenn H. Asquith 978-0-8170-1639-5 $10.00

The Work of the Church Treasurer, Revised Edition Thomas E. McLeod
978-0-8170-1189-5 $13.00

The Work of the Church Trustee Orlando L. Tibbetts 978-0-8170-0825-3 $10.00

The Work of the Clerk, New Edition M. Ingrid Dvirnak 978-0-8170-1253-3 $10.00

The Work of the Deacon & Deaconess, 2nd Revised Edition Harold Nichols
978-0-8170-1755-2 $10.99

The Work of the Pastor Victor D. Lehman 978-0-8170-1473-5 $12.00

Work of the Pastoral Relations Committee Emmett V. Johnson
978-0-8170-0984-7 $11.00

The Work of the Sunday School Superintendent Idris W. Jones, Revised by
Ruth L. Spencer 978-0-8170-1229-8 $10.00

The Work of the Usher Alvin D. Johnson 978-0-8170-0356-2 $10.00

The Work of the Worship Committee Linda Bonn 978-0-8170-1294-6 $10.00

NOW AVAILABLE IN SETS!

- **The Work of the Church Series** 978-0-8170-1487-2 $139.99
  Includes 15 books in the series!

- **The Work of the Church Mini-Set** 978-0-8170-1488-9 $40.00
  The five-book set includes our most popular titles: *The Work of the Deacon
  & Deaconess, The Work of the Usher, The Work of the Sunday School
  Superintendent, The Work of the Church Trustee,* and *The Work of the Pastor.*

**Order online at
www.judsonpress.com
or call 800-458-3766**

JUDSON PRESS
PUBLISHERS SINCE 1824